Psychiatric Presentations in General Practice

A Guide to Holistic Management

SECOND EDITION

Psychiatric Presentations in General Practice

A Guide to Holistic Management

SECOND EDITION

K.S. JACOB
MBBS, DPM, MD, PhD, FRCPsych, FRANZCP
Professor of Psychiatry, Christian Medical College
Vellore, India

ANJU KURUVILLA MBBS, MD
Professor of Psychiatry, Christian Medical College
Vellore, India

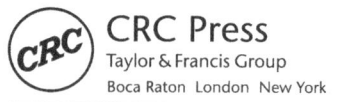

CRC Press
Taylor & Francis Group
Boca Raton London New York

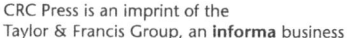

CRC Press is an imprint of the
Taylor & Francis Group, an **informa** business

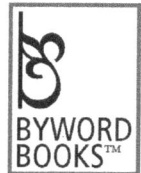

BYWORD
BOOKS™

First edition published by Byword Books Private Limited in 2010

CRC Press
Taylor & Francis Group
6000 Broken Sound Parkway NW, Suite 300
Boca Raton, FL 33487-2742

© 2017 by Taylor & Francis Group, LLC
CRC Press is an imprint of Taylor & Francis Group, an Informa business

No claim to original U.S. Government works

Printed in Great Britain by Ashford Colour Press Ltd
Version Date: 20160816

International Standard Book Number-13: 978-1-4987-6694-4 (Paperback)
International Standard Book Number-13: 978-1-138-72574-4 (Hardback)

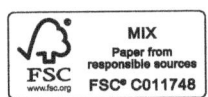

For

Molly and Amita
and
Santosh, Rhea and Lara

for giving us the space to follow our dreams

Contents

SECTION V   Common Clinical Presentations Among Children

SECTION VI   Basic Issues in Management

SECTION VII   Appendix: Information Leaflets

SECTION VIII

Foreword to the Second Edition

It gives me pleasure to introduce to the reader *Psychiatric Presentations in General Practice*, which has proven its value in its return as a second edition. This book addresses the felt need of non-psychiatrists in taking care of psychiatric problems in the general practice and general medical setting. Unlike standard psychiatric textbooks that adopt a theoretical framework to psychiatry, this book's approach grew out of the practical experience of the authors in managing psychiatric problems and teaching junior doctors in the primary and secondary care setting.

The key feature of this book is the approach where practice takes on an important and theoretical value. Of the 10 steps emphasized in this book, only three fall in the standard medical management: history and physical examination, diagnosis, and prescribing medication. The remaining steps go beyond the standard medical approach in emphasizing the role of the patient, the family in their illness, acknowledging their distress, and the therapeutic relationship between the doctor and patient. In enunciating these principles the authors make a theoretical shift from a "diagnosis–drug treatment approach" to a broader framework of "caring for illness," understanding illness in context, and taking care of the sick person. The authors emphasize the value of the instinctive tendency of general practitioners to be wary of disease labels. They further argue that diagnosis should be made more robust by careful discrimination so that the presentation is properly differentiated between distress and disorder. This paradigm shift that integrates a theoretical diagnosis with a broader approach of seeing the sick person in context is essential not only for psychological problems but in every disease. Therein lies the importance of this book.

Normally these steps remain at the sub-theoretical level, learnt by trial and error and long years of experience. Skilled practitioners find it hard to explain what they do in practice to take care of patients and make them get better. The hallmark of a good teacher is to be able to explain what they do in practice. The authors through the "ten-step approach" are able to help others learn their practical approach.

I have found this approach easy to teach to medical students. We have also used this textbook for a distance learning course in family medicine with a supplementary self-learning teaching module.

Today, as practitioners of medicine, we are constrained by evidence-based medicine, doing only what the evidence allows us to do. In stating their approach, the authors emphasize that practice is far bigger than making a criterion-based diagnosis and prescribing an evidence-based treatment. This book encourages all of us to exert our full role as doctors, going beyond the evidence and taking care of the sick person. By opening the door of the theoretical framework, the book encourages doctors in other fields to write down their lessons of practice in a way that can be learnt by other students, teachers, and practitioners.

ANAND ZACHARIAH, MD
Professor of Medicine
Head, Department of Medicine
Christian Medical College
Vellore 632002
Tamil Nadu, India

7 September 2016

Foreword to the First Edition

Mental illness can present in an overt manner, as in the obviously disturbed psychotic patient, or it can be subtle – it shocks close relatives when a suicide occurs. Whatever the presentation, there is a shroud of mystery, suspicion, and a feeling of helplessness, both within society and the primary care physician.

Our medical schools teach us to make accurate diagnosis of the "disease" so that the best "treatment" can be given to the patient. Unfortunately, not everyone who comes to the doctor for help has got a "disease" defined as an organic pathology. Many people have an "illness" defined as symptoms arising from psychosocial distress. Non-organic disease, also referred to as somatization disorders, forms a large component of health problems presenting to physicians at all levels of healthcare. Our individual personalities, cultural and religious beliefs, and social and economic situations determine how we react to the stresses of daily life. Medical doctors, who are not psychiatrists, are poorly equipped to detect psychosocial stress, unless it is very obvious. When non-organic illness is recognized, it is usually after protracted laboratory tests have been done, at much expense, to rule out organic pathology.

This book addresses these blind spots in non-psychiatrist physicians by providing a simple and practical approach to non-organic illness. The question-and-answer format and the 10-point framework is friendly and builds confidence in dealing with unfamiliar aspects of mental health. The format aims to enable doctors to offer patients appropriate treatments, without wading through the pedantic terminology of psychiatric diagnoses.

This fresh, practical, and unique approach will help to demystify psychiatry as a specialty and, in the process, will empower non-psychiatrists to treat mental illness themselves, always recognizing when specialist help is needed. This will serve to ameliorate the huge burden of mental ill health.

ALKA GANESH, MD
Professor of Medicine
Head, Department of Family Medicine
Christian Medical College
Vellore 632002
Tamil Nadu, India

18 November 2009

Preface to the Second Edition

It has been six years since the first edition of *Psychiatric Presentations in General Practice: A Guide to Holistic Management* was published. It was born out of our experience as psychiatrists working in general medical settings, which resulted in the realization that specialist approaches were inappropriate for the complex challenges faced by physicians and general practitioners (GPs) in primary care, in recognizing and treating mental distress and illness. We found that dilution of specialist psychiatric approaches to adapt to primary care did not provide an adequate and appropriate framework for the reality of general and family practice. The "goodness of fit" of this approach was poor.

The differences in settings and perspectives in primary care called for a unique approach; it needed to be one that would suit the context of primary care and its different reality, rather than one imported from tertiary care. Patients who present to physicians in primary care often have non-specific symptoms, mild, mixed, sub-syndromal, and less-than-classical presentations that cluster around the case threshold; this defies formal classification of the condition, making it difficult for physicians to make a diagnosis. The detailed and separate protocols suggested by specialists are also unsuitable for general and family practice. Approaches emphasized by psychiatrists, and seconded by academic GPs, are more suited to tertiary care practice than the reality of primary care. In fact, diluted tertiary care approaches are inapplicable in primary care; this has resulted in family and general practitioners not being able to acquire the required skills to deal effectively with many of their patients, leading to a lack of confidence in this area among such physicians. The consequence has been that physicians, who are unable to diagnose psychiatric disorders in their settings are often unable to treat their patients, using the conventional protocols for psychiatric management.

This book is an outcome of attempts to provide solutions to such dilemmas. It suggests an alternative approach to diagnosis and management, viz. the recognition of broad clinical presentations (delirium, dementia, substance use, psychosis, medically unexplained symptoms, etc.) and common symptomatic protocols for management.

Inspiration and support for adopting such an approach also came from the CMC-Anveshi Collective, a group of professionals working in humanities, social sciences and medicine, who were critiquing medicine and medical practice. The project, which culminated in a book (*Towards a Critical Medical Practice: Reflections on the Dilemmas of Medical Culture Today* by Anand Zachariah, R. Srivatsan and Susie Tharu [eds], Orient Blackswan, New Delhi, 2010), highlighted the need to move out of narrow biomedical models to examine the issues related to mental health, distress, illness, and disease from a much broader, multi-, inter-, and trans-disciplinary framework.

The six years since the publication of the book has also been a time for further reflection on the approach used. General feedback from physicians who have used the approach suggested has been very positive. While the basic approach of the book remains unchanged, the present edition amplifies on the techniques suggested, fills in gaps identified, elaborates on clinical descriptions, provides examples, and discusses controversies. While the 10 steps suggested may appear a little contrived in some situations, they actually reflect principles and practice used by competent physicians and general practitioners. The simple approach allows for easy repetition and practice, thereby enhancing mastery and confidence and increasing patient and physician satisfaction.

We would like to thank Dinesh Sinha and Byword Books, New Delhi, for continued support. We would like to thank our new publishers, Taylor and Francis, for bringing out the Second Edition.

K.S. JACOB
ANJU KURUVILLA

February 2016

Preface to the First Edition

The Department of Psychiatry at the Christian Medical College, Vellore, was established in 1957. The hospital is a short-stay facility for people with mental illness. It is different from most psychiatric facilities in that the patient and the family are admitted and they live in self-contained cottages. The emphasis on educating and empowering the family in addition to treating the person with mental illness allows for holistic care. The fact that families stay with the ill relative also allows for a transfer of skill and confidence in managing problems secondary to the illness, in addition to providing knowledge.

The consultation–liaison service of the department to the primary care facilities, secondary and tertiary hospitals of the Christian Medical College, Vellore, allowed us to experience the reality of general medical settings. Our work and interaction with physicians in non-psychiatric facilities provided insights usually not available to psychiatrists practicing in tertiary and specialist settings.

The Department has had a structured and well-established psychiatric training programme for its medical, nursing and allied health students, and for physicians training in the specialties of general medicine, child health, family and community medicine, physical medicine and rehabilitation, and neurology. The programme has been going on for over four decades and provides a basic introduction to mental disorders and their treatment. It is a good programme by most national and international standards.

And yet, the answer to the question *"Are physicians trained by the department able to manage people with psychiatric disorders in their clinical practice?"* was a resounding "No". At best, most were able to identify the need for psychiatric referral, while a few gained confidence in the use of antidepressant medication. The vast majority were intimidated by the thought of managing psychiatric presentations in their practice and provided less than optimal care.

A diligent analysis of the programme and its impact on physician training suggested that it was employing specialist perspectives and was using psychiatric facilities for training physicians in diagnosing and managing people with mental disorders. These physicians went back to their general hospitals and were not able to diagnose and manage people with psychiatric presentations in their clinical practice.

Our work in non-psychiatric settings taught us that the people who attend specialist facilities differ from those who seek help from non-psychiatric hospitals. Psychiatric presentations in non-psychiatric hospitals were milder, with a mixture of symptoms, making the formal diagnosis difficult. The inability to label the psychiatric syndrome made most physicians unsure as to how to proceed with management. They frequently referred such patients, many of whom refused to attend the psychiatric hospital because of the stigma of mental illness.

Our work in non-specialist settings suggested the need for identifying the broad clinical psychiatric presentations and recognizing common clinical situations where expertise was required. We realized that the need was to transfer skill and confidence, in addition to providing knowledge. We also became conscious that simplifying issues did not mean simple solutions. We understood that modules for managing psychiatric presentations need to be developed using physician perspectives and for the kind of patients who attend general medical settings, rather than by recommending specialist perspectives more suited for managing people with severe and complex disorders who attend tertiary care.

We have developed teaching modules for the e-learning website of the Christian Medical College, Vellore and for the Government of Tamil Nadu's Special Hospital Project. The issues related to problems in managing psychiatric disorders in general medical settings have been published in national and international journals. A recent review of these modules showed that the majority employed very similar and overlapping steps. We realized that the minor variations in these modules also added to the confusion and reduced physician confidence. After a careful analysis of the steps suggested in these modules, we understood that they could be summarized into a common 10-step guide for most presentations and clinical situations. The 10 steps, in addition to the identification of the clinical presentation, the exclusion of organic and medical causes and the symptomatic management, included the need to understand patient perspectives, acknowledge distress, provide education, and support and suggest strategies for coping. It also mandated the need to negotiate a treatment plan. All these steps are part of good clinical practice and they include ingredients for efficient consultation, effective management, and good communication between doctors and their patients.

We would like to thank the many patients who allowed us to understand their problems, appreciate their difficulties, learn from their presentations, see their point of view, and help us comprehend the complexity of the issues. We would like to thank our many non-psychiatric colleagues who allowed us to work in their hospitals and challenged us to look for less complex solutions, simplify protocols, and suggest practical guidelines for use in busy medical and surgical settings. We would like to acknowledge our many psychiatric colleagues who have helped us by using our protocols, suggested improvements in our approach, and commented on the initial drafts of our modules. We would like to thank our publishers for all the support.

This book is a product of many years of work and experience in psychiatric and non-psychiatric settings. It was a humbling experience to know that specialists need to re-examine their solutions while working in different settings.

K.S. JACOB
ANJU KURUVILLA

February 2010

Abbreviations

ADHD	attention deficit hyperactivity disorder
AIDS	acquired immunodeficiency syndrome
CIS-R	Clinical Interview Schedule-Revised
CT	computerized tomography
DSM	Diagnostic and Statistical Manual
ECG	electrocardiogram
EEG	electroencephalogram
ESR	erythrocyte sedimentation rate
GP	general practitioner
HIV	human immunodeficiency virus
ICD	International Classification of Diseases
LFT	liver function tests
MCI	mild cognitive impairment
PLISSIT	Permission, Limited Information, Specific Suggestions, Intensive Therapy
PRN	pro re nata
SSRI	selective serotonin reuptake inhibitor
TSH	thyroid stimulating hormone
UTI	urinary tract infection
WHO	World Health Organization

Section I

Principles

1 The Basic Approach of the Book

The different reality of general hospital settings and primary care make traditional psychiatric concepts, diagnoses, and specific management protocols inappropriate and less useful. The management of psychiatric presentations in general medical settings requires different approaches tailored to local needs and to available perspectives and expertise.

Patients with psychiatric and psychosocial problems who present to primary care and general medical settings differ markedly from those seen in tertiary psychiatric facilities. The former have problems that are milder in severity and have mixed presentations, which cannot be easily identified and labeled using traditional psychiatric diagnoses. The different reality of presentations in primary care makes diagnostic decision-making difficult, and argues strongly for the futility of sub-categorization of psychiatric presentations in general medical settings. While the failure to recognize and label psychiatric disorders in general medical settings has often been blamed on poor education and skills among physicians, psychiatrists who regularly work in primary care appreciate the complexity of the task. These less-than-classical clinical presentations imply that even psychiatrists working in such facilities would misclassify patients, if their diagnostic skills are compared against standardized interview schedules in primary care settings. In addition, the symptomatic nature of all psychiatric treatments means that diagnostic sub-categorization may not be mandatory for management.

On the other hand, general practitioners and physicians working in primary care and medical settings recognize the importance of psychosocial context (e.g. stress, personal resources, coping, social supports, and culture) and their impact on mental health. They prefer not to use mental disorder labels because of the high rates of spontaneous remission and placebo response. They also argue that many people with mild disorders do not improve with antidepressant medication. On the other hand, their symptoms seem to ameliorate with a reduction in psychosocial stress and increased environmental supports. General practitioners are also seriously concerned about the medicalization of all personal and social distress. They argue that the use of symptoms, within the range of normal human emotions, to diagnose mental disorders, without consideration of context, in particular psychosocial hardship, essentially flags non-clinically significant distress, especially at lower degrees of severity.

Consequently, many physicians and general practitioners are uncomfortable with the use of the concepts, categories, and labels of mental disorder, with their disease halo, which sidestep the disease–illness dichotomy while attempting to encompass both disease and distress. (Disease portrays abnormalities of structure and function, while illness is used to represent the subjective experience of suffering.) Therefore, they often do not use psychiatric categories at all, preferring to avoid potentially stigmatizing and meaningless labels. Consequently, the International Classification of Primary Care-2, the standard for general and family practice and primary care, focuses on reasons for clinical encounters, patient data, and clinical activity. In addition, "mixed anxiety depression" and "adjustment disorders" are preferred to the traditional and classical psychiatric categories – major depression and generalized anxiety.

The difficulty in categorization of psychiatric presentations is further compounded by the complex and separate protocols for each traditional psychiatric syndrome. Separate protocols may be neither necessary nor practical for patients who present to primary care. The training of physicians in psychiatry, often set in specialist facilities rather than in primary and secondary care settings, is inappropriate and disempowers physicians. The diluted tertiary care concepts, classifications, and management strategies enforced top down are seldom practiced.

The need for managing psychiatric presentations, mental distress, and disease in primary care and general practice demands an approach that does not sub-categorize psychiatric presentations, includes the use of neutral diagnostic labels, and reduces the stigma associated with psychiatric labels. The approach advocated in this book argues that clinical presentation be treated without labels. Though such an approach goes against general medical tradition, it is worthwhile, as the mixed nature of presentations seen in primary care and arbitrary divisions make psychiatric classification much less meaningful. The minor variations in presentation do not warrant major changes in the treatment approach. All common presentations of psychiatric morbidity (i.e. dementia, delirium, substance use, psychosis, and common mental disorders) have common themes in treatment. An amalgamation of these common issues, specifically suited for primary care, has been attempted in this book. The general principles in assessment and management are enumerated.

This book is a practical guide to common mental health problems encountered in general medical practice. It includes simple guidelines and a systematic approach to identifying, assessing, and managing such problems in adults and children. The book incorporates patient information leaflets, as well as guidelines for the doctor as to when patients must be referred to a psychiatrist for specialist management. The book is meant for medical, nursing and paramedical students, general practitioners, non-psychiatric physicians, and counselors.

2 The Context of Primary Care and General Hospital Settings

The context of primary care and general practice settings differ from that seen in psychiatric and specialist care. Patients with psychiatric disorders who attend general medical settings usually have milder illness with mixed symptom presentations, often associated with psychosocial stress. On the other hand, patients attending psychiatric centers often present with severe, chronic, and complex conditions. Physicians, general and family practitioners, also employ differing concepts and frameworks to those used by specialists. Consequently, it is difficult to apply the traditional diagnostic classification and categories to clinical practice in primary and secondary hospital settings. In addition, the specific and detailed management protocols recommended by specialist psychiatric perspectives, although adapted to primary care, are detailed, cumbersome, impractical, and inappropriate for routine use. There is a need to employ physician perspectives, which are applicable in general medical settings. The focus should also be on the transfer of skill and confidence rather than the passive acquisition of knowledge.

INTRODUCTION

Primary care, and general and family practice settings differ from psychiatric and specialist facilities in a variety of ways. The kind of patients who visit these facilities and their clinical presentations also vary markedly from the people who are treated in specialist settings. This chapter discusses these issues in detail.

WHAT IS THE PREVALENCE OF PSYCHIATRIC DISORDERS IN PRIMARY CARE?

Many investigations have established the prevalence of common psychiatric problems in primary care, and general and family practice in many parts of the world. Numerous studies have also documented depression, anxiety, and common mental disorders in general hospital settings. The estimates for the prevalence of such presentations have ranged from 10% to 50% of patients attending primary care, with an average of about a quarter to a third suffering from such conditions.

WHY DOES THE PREVALENCE OF PSYCHIATRIC CONDITIONS DIFFER ACROSS REGIONS?

There are many reasons for differences in prevalence of psychiatric disorders in primary care across regions. Clinical presentations and the meaning they hold for people differ across regions and cultures. Idioms of distress and beliefs about illness and suffering vary across societies resulting in differing presentations. People from non-western cultures are said to somatize their emotional distress (i.e. selectively focus on somatic accompaniments of distress rather than highlight emotional reactions). Their cultures tend to focus on somatic symptoms even while acknowledging emotional stress. Local and traditional systems of medicine also selectively offer particular physical explanations for emotional reactions cementing such beliefs and increasing the probability of such presentations. In addition, physicians practicing in these regions also preferentially focus on somatic symptoms, resulting in their more frequent elicitation. The belief that physicians are experts in managing physical disease means that even people with emotional distress will seek help from primary care for the somatic accompaniments of psychological reactions. Differences in help-seeking for emotional distress varies across regions, resulting in variations in prevalence.

WHAT ARE THE STRATEGIES CURRENTLY EMPLOYED IN PRIMARY CARE?

The high prevalence of these psychiatric disorders, the magnitude of disability and distress, and the shortage of psychiatrists and specialists have focused efforts on managing them within the context of primary care. Consequently, educating general and family practitioners, preparing practice guidelines, and conducting courses to improve the practitioners' clinical skills have been attempted. The World Health Organization (WHO) has developed algorithms to make diagnoses easier. They have also developed simple assessment guidelines and recommended protocols for the management of such presentations in primary care. These efforts resulted in the expectation that depression would be managed in primary care.

WHAT ARE THE RECOGNITION AND TREATMENT RATES IN PRIMARY CARE?

Despite such expectations, the detection rate for depression and common mental disorders in general practice and primary care continues to be low. Despite piloting, field studies, and acceptance by academic general practitioners, the watered down psychiatric approach, when employed in primary care, has few takers in actual practice. Many physicians find the numerous case-finding instruments and screening questionnaires to diagnose individual mental disorders too cumbersome and time-consuming for routine use. The many diagnostic criteria for individual psychiatric disorders are elaborate and difficult to apply in routine and busy general medical practice. Detailed treatment guidelines also do not seem to improve management.

Consequently, low recognition and treatment rates in primary care persist despite repeated exhortation to improve clinical practice. The culture of psychiatry in primary care borrows heavily from academic and tertiary care psychiatry and attempts to adapt it to the reality of primary care. The compromise is uneasy, unstable, and difficult to apply in general practice.

WHAT ARE THE COMMON PSYCHIATRIC AND PSYCHOSOCIAL PROBLEMS SEEN IN PRIMARY CARE?

The most common clinical presentation of psychiatric problems in primary care is one of physical symptoms, without medical explanations. Such presentations are often called unexplained physical symptoms, unexplained somatic symptoms, medically unexplained physical symptoms, medically unexplained symptoms, chronic fatigue, fibromyalgia, neurasthenia, etc. Many patients with medically unexplained complaints also have symptoms of anxiety and depression. Such presentations include excessive and distressing concern for symptoms (i.e. called "health anxiety") or people with such presentations also have disabling common mental disorders (i.e. anxiety and depressive syndromes). The other presentations seen include delirium, dementia, substance use and dependence, and psychoses. The failure to recognize and manage such common psychiatric disorders has a major impact on help-seeking and healthcare delivery.

WHAT HAPPENS TO PATIENTS WHO DO NOT GET HELP FROM PHYSICIANS?

The absence of physical causes for medically unexplained symptoms often results in the physician downplaying their importance or ignoring the distress. Physicians, because of their training, often selectively focus on the physical complaints of their patients and frequently ignore psychological symptoms. Their competence in treating physical complaints and their lack of confidence in managing emotional distress and psychological reactions decides their focus. Consequently, many patients are often dissatisfied with the medical care they receive and often shop for different treatments, visiting diverse facilities involved in healthcare and healing.

Those with delirium, dementia, and psychosis who are not recognized in medical settings also shop for treatments, and the delay in starting treatment often proves costly. Those with substance use and dependence who are not identified will continue their habit to the detriment of their health, their families, and communities.

IF PSYCHIATRIC PRESENTATIONS ARE SO COMMON IN PRIMARY CARE, WHY IS IT DIFFICULT TO RECOGNIZE AND MANAGE THESE IN CLINICAL PRACTICE?

There are many reasons for discomfort among physicians in managing psychiatric disorders in primary care. These include:

- Medical teaching programs for physicians:
  - Usually focus on the classical cases with definite physical signs and underlying medical causes
  - Rarely discuss patients with medically unexplained symptoms
- Psychiatric training programs are based in specialist settings, and employ complex psychiatric perspectives and management strategies:
  - Usually focus on classical syndromes, and severe and chronic conditions rather than milder and mixed presentations of non-specific symptoms
  - Usually promote the acquisition of knowledge rather than skills and confidence in managing these conditions.

WHAT ARE THE TRADITIONAL EXPLANATIONS OFFERED FOR THE LACK OF SKILLS IN THE DIAGNOSIS AND MANAGEMENT OF PSYCHIATRIC DISORDERS BY GENERAL PHYSICIANS?

The lack of knowledge of psychiatric disorders and their treatment, absence of motivation to learn among students, lack of time in busy medical and surgical settings, and lack of transfer of skills during basic medical training are mentioned as possible reasons. The inferior standard of psychiatry teaching and vagueness of the subject are also listed as possible explanations.

ARE THERE OTHER EXPLANATIONS?

Physicians and psychiatrists who work in primary and secondary care settings would argue that psychiatrists who usually work in tertiary and specialist facilities do not understand the reality of medical settings. They fail to comprehend the needs of the patients who visit, nor the clinicians who work in such facilities. They also highlight the fact that most training programs in psychiatry for physicians employ specialist perspectives, psychiatric jargon, diagnoses, and labels which are difficult to apply in primary care; complex treatment protocols are taught which, while satisfying the needs of psychiatrists, are not appropriate for physicians working in primary and secondary care. The focus of most psychiatric training programs for physicians is psychiatric theory and knowledge rather than the acquisition of skill and confidence in managing psychiatric presentations.

WHAT ARE THE DIFFERENCES BETWEEN PATIENTS ATTENDING A PSYCHIATRIC HOSPITAL AND THOSE WHO PRESENT TO PRIMARY CARE?

The many differences are listed in Table 2.1. These differences in settings demand different approaches to management. They mandate the use of strategies and protocols developed in primary care rather than specialist protocols adapted for use in general practice.

WHAT ARE THE GENERAL TRENDS IN MEDICINE THAT IMPACT CLINICAL CARE?

Recent trends have had a significant impact on general practice and primary care. These include specialization within medicine, medicalization of distress, and standardization of diagnosis for insurance reimbursement.

The growth of medicine, particularly tertiary care, over the past century has resulted in the decline of family medicine and general practice. This reduction has been inversely proportional to the spectacular rise of specialist approaches. Many problems of patients presenting to general physicians and family practitioners are now viewed from a specialist perspective. This is true across all medical disciplines and particularly true of psychiatric disorders in primary care.

The second development, which has significantly affected the identification and treatment of psychiatric presentations in primary care is the progressive medicalization of all personal and social distress. This has lowered thresholds for the tolerance of mild symptoms and for seeking medical attention for such complaints. Patients visit GPs when they are disturbed or distressed, when they are in pain or are worried about the implication of their symptoms. However, the provision of psychological and social support currently mandates the need for medical models, labels and treatments to justify medical input.

The insurance based medical systems, common across capitalistic countries,

TABLE 2.1

The Differences between Mental Disorders Presenting to Psychiatric and General Medical Settings

Characteristic	Psychiatric facility	General medical setting
Severity of illness	Usually severe	Often mild
Complexity of problem	Usually complex	Often simple
Chronicity of condition	Usually chronic	Often brief
Distinct/mixed presentation	Distinct and classical syndromes	Mixed presentation common
Psychosocial adversity	May be present	Often correlated
Motivation to seek psychiatric treatment	Present	May be absent
Predictors of outcome	Genetic and disease predictors important	Psychosocial predictors usually important
Availability and expertise of doctors	Specialist expertise available	Physician perspective and expertise available
Concepts and framework	Psychiatric	Physician
Focus	Presenting syndrome	Patient context
Use of psychotropic medication	Common and in higher dose	Rare, prefer psychosocial interventions
Cost: Time and money	Usually prolonged consultations	Often brief and inexpensive

demands standardized and uniform practice for reimbursement of medical expenses. Consequently, psychiatry now employs symptom counts to improve diagnostic reliability. The complete discounting of the patient's context (e.g. stress, personality, coping, supports, etc.) means that while the reliability of psychiatric diagnosis has increased, its validity remains questionable. In addition, there is marked heterogeneity within diagnostic heads. On the other hand, psychiatric treatment remains essentially symptomatic and not directly linked to diagnosis.

CONCLUSION

The context of primary care and general medical settings, and the major differences between them and tertiary and specialist psychiatric facilities demand a different approach to the diagnosis and management of psychiatric disorders. The differences in clinical presentations mandate the need to tailor primary care approaches to the patients rather than employ specialist perspectives, which are inappropriate for the local needs.

BOX 2.1 SOME DIFFERENCES BETWEEN PSYCHIATRIC APPROACHES AND GENERAL PRACTICE PERSPECTIVES

Recent psychiatric classifications have focused on improving the reliability of psychiatric diagnosis. The absence of laboratory markers and pathognomonic symptoms and the use of symptoms, within the normal range of human emotions, for diagnosis has forced psychiatry to concentrate on the clinical syndrome, i.e. a collection of symptoms. Consequently, psychiatric diagnoses are symptom counts sans context. The discounting of context implies a reduced emphasis on personality, stress, environmental supports, culture, and coping, making it difficult to separate normal human distress from mental disorders. The term disorder sidesteps the disease–illness controversy including both disease and illness. Consequently, psychiatric labels medicalize personal and social distress.

On the other hand, physicians recognize the importance of psychosocial context (e.g. stress, personal resources, coping, social supports, and culture) and their effect on mental health. They prefer not to use mental disorder labels because of the high rates of spontaneous remission and placebo response and the absence of improvement with antidepressant medication in those with mild disorders. General practitioners are seriously concerned about the medicalization of all personal and social distress. They argue that the use of symptoms to diagnose mental disorders, without consideration of context, in particular psychosocial hardship, essentially flags non-clinically significant distress, especially at lower degrees of severity.

Many physicians and general practitioners are uncomfortable with the use of the concept of mental disorder, with its disease halo. They often do not use psychiatric categories at all, preferring to avoid potentially stigmatizing and meaningless labels. Consequently, the International Classification of Primary Care-2, focuses on reasons for clinical encounters, patient data, and clinical activity.

Context and local knowledge are critical to understanding illness in primary care. Universal abstractions may not fit local reality and may artificially force structures. Primary care should be able to choose a different framework for the management of psychiatric and emotional problems. Contexts should not only change medical practice, but also be able to change medical perspectives.

The complexity of the issues related to the diagnosis and management of such presentations demands a re-evaluation of the issues. Alternative approaches have to be rooted in primary care for them to be useful and successfully employed.

3 Diagnosis and Management of Psychiatric Presentations in General Medical Settings

The differences between the context of primary care and general hospital settings, on the one hand, and tertiary care psychiatric facilities on the other, demand a re-evaluation of the approaches to diagnosing and managing patients with psychosocial and psychiatric problems. This chapter discusses the approach to diagnosis and management of psychiatric presentations in primary care. It discusses the theoretical basis and emphasizes the practical issues related to such an approach. It also contrasts the method to traditional psychiatric thought and practice.

The use of clinical presentations without formal psychiatric diagnosis and the symptomatic management of people with such presentations in primary care are complementary. These approaches describe the current practice among competent physicians working in primary care. The common protocol includes the identification of the clinical presentation, the exclusion and management of medical and organic causes, and symptomatic management of psychiatric symptoms. It also includes acknowledging distress, eliciting patient perspectives, education about disease and illness, suggesting general and specific coping strategies, negotiating participation and responsibility in treatment, and giving an appointment for review.

INTRODUCTION

Psychiatric concepts and framework form the basis of primary care psychiatry, albeit diluted and modified to meet general and family practice settings. However, such a top-down approach is unsuitable for medical settings and disempowers physicians. The failure to recognize the classical psychiatric syndromes in populations with milder and mixed presentations does not allow the physician to make a diagnosis impeding management. The issues are discussed.

WHAT IS THE TRADITIONAL PSYCHIATRIC APPROACH TO DIAGNOSIS?

The lack of pathognomonic symptoms for psychiatric disorders and the absence of gold standards and laboratory tests for diagnosis of psychiatric conditions forced psychiatrists to focus on clinical presentations. However, the use of relatively limited repertoire of human emotional responses, individual perception of unpleasant feelings, and phenomena within the normal range of emotions meant that disorders were defined around clinical syndromes (rather than individual symptoms). Psychiatric syndromes are a cluster of symptoms, which result in disturbance in cognition, emotional regulation, and behavior; they disrupt functioning and produce clinically significant distress.

Nevertheless, the use of clinical syndromes without a standard approach to diagnosis frequently resulted in diagnostic disagreements even among psychiatrists. The classificatory movement within psychiatry decided to focus on symptom counts to increase the reliability of psychiatric diagnosis. Such symptom counts, while improving inter-rater reliability, also meant that the varied contexts, which demand interpretation by clinicians, were discounted. In addition, the dimension between normal reactions and psychopathological states mean arbitrary categorical divisions.

The discounting of stress and context makes it difficult to separate normal human distress from mental disorders. Consequently, psychiatric labels medicalize mental distress. Stress and trauma – acute (e.g. bereavement), recurrent (e.g. domestic violence), or chronic (e.g. poverty); physical disease and disability; interpersonal difficulties; and other social determinants are associated with symptoms of depression and anxiety. There is evidence to suggest that mental distress and illness are linked to social determinants of health. The failure to meet basic needs (e.g. clean water, sanitation, nutrition, housing, and immunization) due to poverty impacts mental health. Patriarchy results in gross gender injustice and significantly affects the health of girls and women. Low education and unemployment are common causes of mental distress. Structural violence, discrimination, social exclusion, political oppression, ethnic cleansing, and forced migration are common in poor countries. Armed conflicts and war take their toll. These risk factors for poor mental health work through insecurity, hopelessness, rapid social change, risk of violence, and poor physical health.

Consequently, the clinically and statistically significant relationship between psychosocial adversity and mental ill-health (i.e. distress, illness, and disease) complicates the simplistic "atheoretical" approach to psychiatric diagnosis. Current psychiatric classifications provide labels by arbitrarily dividing the many complex dimensions of mental health, distress, illness, and disease into dichotomous normal/ abnormal (disorder) categories. The discipline with its biomedical framework transfers the disease halo, reserved for severe mental illness, to all psychiatric diagnoses. It locates primary pathology in the individual when causal mechanism can lie in the environment. Medication-based solutions for problems of living are controversial.

Nevertheless, mental health, particularly in low- and middle-income countries, is often addressed through urgency-driven medical solutions, which are preferred to public health approaches. Public health is reduced to biomedical model. Primary care is mistaken for public health, and the focus is on outreach clinics rather than a concerted multisectoral public health response (i.e. provision of basic needs, health care, employment, justice, etc.)

How does the absence of laboratory symptoms impact diagnosis?

The lack of laboratory diagnosis, the absence of pathognomonic symptoms for specific categories, and the problems in eliciting individual symptoms has resulted in the use of a collection of symptoms (syndrome) for diagnosis. Nevertheless, such clinical syndromes are often heterogeneous in etiology, pathology, clinical features, treatment response, prognosis, course, and outcome. The many operational criteria and the numerous revisions of the classificatory systems often give psychiatric diagnoses an aura and equate the many categories with physical diseases. Yet, psychiatric categories can convey little information about etiology, treatment, and prognosis, and often create a spurious impression of understanding.

Diseases are essentially professional conceptualizations. They often assume biological dysfunction and disadvantage. Many psychiatric categories are also based on a social concept of agreed undesirability. Such conceptualizations are preferred to viewpoints, which argue for sin (from a religious point of view), crime (by the law), or social problem (from a social work perspective). Illness, on the other hand, is a sociocultural construction of sickness as perceived and experienced by the patient. Recent psychiatric classifications have employed the term "disorder" as a compromise, sidestepping the disease–illness controversy.

WHAT IS THE CONCEPTUAL APPROACH TO MENTAL DISORDERS?

An understanding of the psychiatric models, concepts and framework of diagnosis, classification, and treatment is critical prior to a critique of psychiatric disorders in general practice and primary care. Psychiatric disorders have been viewed through many conceptual frameworks: psychological and psychoanalytical; cognitive and behavioral; social, moral, and religious frameworks; and the medical model. However, the medical model has increased its hold on psychiatric theory over the latter half of the twentieth century.

The medical model views psychiatric disorders as diseases, presumes central nervous system etiology and pathogenesis, records signs and symptoms, proposes differential diagnoses, employs somatic therapies, and prognosticates about course and outcome. The recognition of likely neurotransmitter mechanisms and the response to particular pharmacological medications in patients with severe mental disorders have reinforced the conviction that disorders such as severe depression, especially for the sub-groups with bipolar disorders, psychotic symptoms, stupor, and melancholic features, are a disease of the brain.

The speculation and theories about biological abnormalities in the brain for psychiatric disorders have not directly been proved. While people with severe mental disorders seem to differ from normal individuals on some biochemical parameters, these differences are not specific for these conditions nor do they allow for clear separation and consequent use as diagnostic laboratory tests to confirm these conditions. Nevertheless, psychiatrists argue the successful treatment with pharmaceutical medication, with their specific mechanisms of action, support biological etiology of psychiatric conditions. However, the marked variability of response to medication, the variability of course, and outcome of disorders and treatment-resistant disorders suggest that the issues are complex and currently unfathomable. Proposing simple neurochemical abnormalities as causal for complex behaviors is not only inadequate on the ground but also philosophically untenable.

As an example, the problems of using a pure medical model for depression with its biological approaches and its limitations in primary care are briefly discussed. Depression seen in primary care is heterogeneous. Psychiatric classifications have many types of depression: can be secondary to medical conditions (e.g. hypothyroidism, diabetes mellitus, and carcinoma pancreas), complicate substance dependence, and due to insight in people with psychosis. Depression can also present as distinct subtypes: melancholia, chronic depression, and as a reaction to severe stress.

Patients present with depressive symptoms precipitated by acute stress (adjustment disorders) and with chronic depression due to multiple stressors and/or due to poor coping skills (dysthymia/chronic and persistent depression). People with a family history of depression can also present with severe melancholia and psychotic depression. However, the use of symptom counts to diagnose depression sans context means that the category depression employed in primary care and the label major depression includes markedly different patterns of illness. While melancholia requires pharmacological interventions, people with chronic depression benefit from long-term psychotherapy and counseling while those with adjustment disorders secondary to severe stress require psychological support. Even though the validity and specific disease status for many labels in the classificatory system (Diagnostic and Statistical Manual [DSM] 5 and International Classification of Diseases [ICD] 10) are not established, the authority and use of the medical model implies otherwise. Accordingly, the disease halo reserved for the more severe forms of depression is also conferred on people with depressive symptoms secondary to stress and poor coping.

Antidepressants have become the treatment of choice for all categories of depression. There is neither the need to speculate on the role of the precipitating stress and coping strategies, nor the requirement to manage them with psychological therapies. The ease of prescribing medication and the investment of time and effort required for cognitive therapy means that psychological intervention is often praised, but seldom practiced. Antidepressants have become the panacea for loneliness, relationship difficulties, interpersonal conflicts, inability to cope with day-to-day stress, and the like. The medicalization of distress is complete.

Another significant issue, especially in the western world, is the role of mental health professionals in managing people with mental illness and distress. Many people with distressing social situations and life events present with symptoms of depression and receive psychiatric labels. Consequently, the mental health team provides the psychological and social supports, which were previously provided by the family and local community. However, the provision of such support by mental health professionals mandates the need for medical models, labels, and treatments to justify medical input. Insurance reimbursement also necessitates the use of disease labels. Consequently, psychiatric culture now tends to view all depression and distress through the disease/medical lens.

The majority of patients who present with depression in primary care have mild symptoms and associated psychosocial stress factors, and are dependent on the availability of personal resources and social supports for recovery. The use of the medical model of depression, which employs symptom counts and refuses to acknowledge the role of context, stress, personality, and coping, may be less appropriate in primary care.

How does the general practitioner's perspective differ from specialist interpretation?

The general practitioner's (GP's) perspective differs from that espoused by a psychiatrist. People with depressive symptoms often present to GPs. Patients visit GPs when they are disturbed or distressed, when they are in pain or worried about the implications of their symptoms. Bereavement, marital discord, inability to cope at work, and financial problems can also lead people to seek help. The difficulty in separating distress from depression becomes a major issue. While psychiatrists suggest that brief screening instruments can easily identify people with depression, most GPs would argue that many of those identified are distressed. The depression GPs encounter is often viewed as secondary to personal and social stress, lifestyle choices or as a product of habitual maladaptive patterns of behavior. Consequently, GPs often hold psychological and social models for depression.

Most GPs and physicians working in primary care accept the medical model of depression during discussions with psychiatrists and academic GPs. However, low detection and treatment rates suggest that the majority subscribe to non-medical, social, and psychological perspectives. Resolution of social adversity, the presence of social supports, and the person's psychological resources seem to have a greater impact on outcome than medical solutions. Antidepressants and short-term counseling do help certain patients. Nevertheless, they are not the answer for all "depression". The difficulty in separating disease from distress and the absence of effective medical solutions for "depression" in primary care are often the compelling reasons for the reluctance of GPs to accept the medical model of depression.

Mixed Presentations in General Practice: Difficulty in Separating Anxiety from Depression

The differences in concepts, perspectives, and frameworks between psychiatry and general/family practice is based on the differences in settings. Psychiatrists practice in specialist settings and see different sub-groups of patients compared to physicians working in primary care. Patients presenting with non-specific symptoms, milder complaints and mixed presentations are routine in primary care. This section highlights the differences between the two settings, which might explain the divergence in perspectives with regard to anxiety and depression. These differences include the following:

- Patients who visit psychiatric facilities often have severe, complex, and chronic illness, and are highly motivated to receive specialist treatment. On the other hand, those who visit GPs have less severe and less distinct forms of illness, with concomitant psychosocial stress.
- Differing conceptual models and perceptions are employed in different settings. Psychiatrists employ medical models while GPs focus on the psychosocial context, stress, personality, and coping.

- In patients attending primary care, symptom scores on standardized interview schedules (e.g. Clinical Interview Schedule-Revised [CIS-R]) are distributed continuously with no point of rarity between cases and non-cases, making dichotomous clinical decision-making difficult.
- Patients in primary care often present with a mixture of symptoms of anxiety and depression.
- Many patients who cross the case threshold do not have the full syndrome attributes of depression or anxiety.
- Labeling of patients with sub-syndromal presentations based on distress and impairment essentially implies a lowering of the threshold for diagnosis.
- Studies using statistical techniques have failed to show superiority of the two-factor anxiety–depression models over the one-factor solution. In addition, the anxiety and depression factors of the two-factor model have always been highly correlated.
- The commonest presentation of psychiatric problems in primary care is with medically unexplained somatic symptoms. However, a significant number of such patients also mention the concomitant presence of psychological stress or distress.
- Etiology of medically unexplained somatic symptoms is unclear. The general tendency is to assume psychogenesis. However, the label "somatization" actually acknowledges medical ignorance rather than understanding.
- Numerous categories of depression in ICD 10 for use in psychiatric settings have been clubbed into a single category of depression in the ICD 10 for primary care. This results in patients with features of biological depression being clubbed with normal people with adjustment reactions due to stress and those who cannot cope with the demands of life because of poor coping skills.
- Many studies have shown a high rate of spontaneous remission of depression and common mental disorders in primary care. The literature on major depression also supports the argument that there is a high rate of spontaneous remission.
- Many authors have highlighted the high rate of improvement in the placebo arms of randomized trials employed to test the efficacy of antidepressant medication.
- Despite efforts at simplification, the guidelines for managing common medical disorders in primary care have proposed elaborate and separate protocols for each of the traditional psychiatric categories, making them impractical for routine use.

Mixed presentations, and the difficulty in separating anxiety from depression in primary care make labels like "mixed anxiety depression" popular among physicians and GPs. Stress related distress, common in primary care, suggest labels like adjustment disorders. Presentations with physical symptoms without medical abnormalities argue for the label "medically unexplained symptoms". Specific presentations associated with stress and poor coping get labels like "tension headache", atypical chest pain, and dyspepsia.

WHAT IS THE BASIS OF PSYCHIATRIC TREATMENT?

Psychiatric treatments are essentially symptomatic. For example, tricyclic antidepressants and serotonin, and norepinephrine-specific reuptake inhibitors work through blocking the reuptake of monoamine neurotransmitters in the synapse, thereby increasing availability. Nevertheless, their action is useful in a variety of conditions. They are employed for depression secondary to medical and organic conditions, as well as for depression in schizophrenia, affective disorders, stress-related conditions and personality disorders. They are also used in a variety of anxiety disorders including panic, phobia, obsessive–compulsive disorder, generalized anxiety, and post-traumatic stress. This is also true for psychological treatment concepts and techniques, which are employed across psychiatric categories. Consequently, while a diagnosis will provide a label, it is a detailed assessment of the patient's current status, which is crucial for management. Such use of specific pharmacological medication and psychotherapeutic techniques across diagnostic categories argues for the lack of diagnostic specificity and for symptomatic use.

WHAT APPROACH WOULD BE SUITED TO PRIMARY CARE?

The differences between patients attending primary care and specialist settings mandate the need for approaches based on and developed in primary care. Two alternative and complementary approaches, rooted in primary care, are suggested:

(i) Management of clinical presentations without a formal diagnosis
(ii) The use of common protocols.

CAN WE MANAGE A CLINICAL PRESENTATION WITHOUT A FORMAL DIAGNOSIS?

The different reality of presentations in primary care makes diagnostic decision-making difficult and argues strongly for the futility of sub-categorization of psychiatric presentations in primary care.

WHAT ARE THE ADVANTAGES OF MANAGING CLINICAL PRESENTATIONS WITHOUT A FORMAL DIAGNOSIS?

The advantages of an approach that does not sub-categorize psychiatric presentations of anxiety, depression, and medically unexplained symptoms in primary care include:

- Use of neutral diagnostic labels reduces the stigma associated with psychiatric terms. Terms such as "functional somatic symptoms" and "medically unexplained symptoms" more accurately describe such cases and should be preferred to "somatization", which rewords the same phenomenon in psychiatric jargon
- Avoids the distress/disease controversy
- Avoids the threshold debate separating distress and disease
- Avoids identification of multiple diagnostic heads due to the high correlation between traditional categories
- Focuses on a holistic approach rather than a symptom checklist.

WHAT ARE THE OTHER CLINICAL PRESENTATIONS WHERE SUCH AN APPROACH CAN BE USED?

Similarly, the identification of other clinical presentations without formal sub-categorization into the traditional psychiatric syndromes is useful. The clinical presentations discussed in this book are:

- *Delirium* – This is a syndrome resulting from a variety of medical and neurological causes. Its clinical presentation is characterized by an acute confusional state in which the patient is disoriented to time, place, and person. It is more frequently seen in the elderly, in patients in intensive care units and during the postoperative period.
- *Dementia* – This is a syndrome characterized by chronic memory loss associated with other cognitive deficits, including aphasia, agnosia, apraxia, difficulty with complex attention, problems with new learning, deficits in social cognition, and loss of executive function. It is often seen in the elderly and is progressive, with social and occupational impairment. Many medical and neurological diseases are causal.
- *Substance Use and Dependence* – These are common clinical presentations and need to be specifically managed. The common substances of use and dependence include alcohol, cannabis, benzodiazepines, and occasionally, opioids. The complications of substance dependence also demand a specific approach to their management.
- *Psychosis* is a clinical presentation characterized by strange beliefs not in keeping with the local culture, hallucinations (auditory and visual), and grossly abnormal behavior. Traditionally, psychoses have been divided into organic, schizophrenia, bipolar, and delusional disorders. While the identification of medical and neurological causes of psychosis is cardinal for treatment, subdivision of the other functional psychoses is not an immediate need in the general medical setting. Such subdivision is also difficult for reasons discussed earlier.
- *Somatic Symptoms* are commonly seen in medical and surgical practice and are detailed separately.
- *Deliberate Self-Harm* – Patients who attempt suicide and harm themselves deliberately are a specific group whose particular needs are discussed in detail.
- *Sexual Dysfunction* is much more common than realized and is very often not recognized in practice; its diagnosis and management are discussed separately.

These presentations lend themselves to such management, as they are a collection of symptoms (syndromes). Their overall management is possible without further sub-categorization, as the treatments in psychiatry are essentially symptomatic. The focus on the few major presentations that have important implications on management will allow the physician to narrow down the management options and choose the correct protocol for therapy. The approach advocated here argues that the symptom presentation be treated without specific diagnostic category labels. While not conforming to medical tradition, this approach recognizes the broad clinical presentation, which is more suitable for use in primary care.

How can a single general protocol for management be used?

The difficulty in the categorization of psychiatric presentations is further compounded by the complex and separate management protocols for each traditional psychiatric syndrome. Separate protocols may not be necessary for patients who present to primary care, nor are they practical in such settings. Minor variations in presentations do not warrant major changes in the treatment approach. All common presentations of non-psychotic psychiatric morbidity have common themes in treatment. An amalgamation of these common issues specifically suited for primary care has been attempted and

---

BOX 3.1 PREFERRED LABELS FOR MENTAL DISTRESS AND ILLNESS IN PRIMARY CARE

Many physicians and general practitioners are uncomfortable with the use of mental disorder labels, as they imply disease. They prefer to avoid potentially stigmatizing and meaningless labels, which essentially flag personal and social distress. They use the International Classification of Primary Care-2 for diagnosis, which focuses on reasons for clinical encounters, patient data, and clinical activity. They also prefer labels such as mixed anxiety and depression to highlight non-specific symptoms, milder and mixed presentations rather than use the traditional psychiatric categories of major depressive disorder and generalized anxiety disorder. While many studies in primary care have documented a high prevalence of mixed anxiety and depression, psychiatry refuses to accept the validity of the category, which is not currently listed in any psychiatric classification.

"Mixed anxiety depression" and "adjustment disorders" are preferred to the traditional psychiatric categories major depression and generalized anxiety. GPs understand the need for psychological support when people are faced with psychosocial adversity.

---

general principles have been enumerated. The following is an example of a general protocol, which has identified the essence of treatment, often useful in patients presenting with common mental disorders to primary care:

- Identify the clinical presentation
- Acknowledge distress
- Elicit the patient's and the family's perspective on symptoms
- Take a focused history; carry out physical examination and laboratory investigations
- Educate the patient and family about illness and treatment
- Prescribe medication
- Discuss the role of stress as a cause and consequence of illness
- Elicit coping strategies
- Transfer responsibility for improvement
- Give an appointment for review.

These steps do not follow any specific theory but are eclectic and address specific concerns of patients who present to primary care and who often receive psychiatric labels.

WHAT ARE THE ADVANTAGES OF A SINGLE GENERAL PROTOCOL?

The advantages of a single protocol include the following: (i) It has a greater chance of mastery and consequent use in clinical practice; (ii) It encourages a holistic approach to care; (iii) The flexible format allows incorporation of specific techniques; (iv) It allows for the treatment of the classic syndrome(s).

While specialists recommend the use of specific treatments, the limited applicability of such protocols in busy general practice settings argues against such approaches. The current psychiatric treatment strategies, despite their elaborate specifications, are essentially symptomatic. Simplifying protocols will ensure their use in routine clinical practice. There is a need to identify such optimal general protocols, and to test their efficacy and effectiveness in clinical practice using randomized controlled trials.

THE PRACTICE–THEORY GAP

It is generally believed that theory drives practice. This is a simplistic interpretation of ground realities. In fact, practice defines theory. The distinction between justice and law is an example. Justice is an agreed concept/value, which is implemented through law. However, the laws often fall short of delivering justice and need to be constantly interpreted and rewritten to provide justice. Similarly, the relief of distress among patients who attend primary care is an agreed aim. It is implemented through different practice guidelines. Many of these recommendations fall short of the ideal and need to be re-examined and reworked. This is particularly true of the diagnosis and management of common mental disorders in primary care. The challenge of relieving emotional distress is currently addressed by practice guidelines based on the medical model. The many issues raised suggest that the current medical diagnostic and therapeutic approaches, which demand sub-categorization and the use of specific treatment protocols, do not meet the challenge and are inappropriate for the task. There is a need to rework the details, keeping in mind the complex nature of the issues.

THE FUTURE

The approaches suggested need to be evaluated as all interventions need an evidence base before implementation in clinical practice. The framework suggested does not at present have an evidence base to support its use in primary care. However, competent clinicians working in primary care already employ similar approaches, which provides for face and content validity. Nevertheless, randomized controlled trials should be employed to prove the efficacy and effectiveness of these approaches. The current medical model places an ideological bar on the discussion of alternative approaches. There is a need for an alternative framework. There is an urgency to narrow the practice–theory gap.

CONCLUSION

The strategies suggested here are based on the argument that it is difficult to sub-categorize clinical presentations of common mental disorders in primary care, and that current psychiatric treatments are essentially symptomatic and are delivered across diagnostic categories. This argument supports the contention that the presentations currently labeled anxiety, depression, or common mental disorders in primary care are illness experiences that do not require disease labels. It makes a case for the provision of support without medicalizing the issues. It also suggests that the standards for medical practice should be based on the issues as seen in primary care rather than those employed in tertiary care and specialist settings.

The focus on clinical presentations without diagnosis and the symptomatic management of people with emotional distress who present to primary care are complementary. These approaches are not new and describe the current practice among competent physicians in primary care. Recent concepts and interventions, based on specialist perspectives, have not only complicated the issues but have disempowered GPs with psychiatric jargon and techniques, which are impractical and counterproductive in primary care settings. The reality of primary care and its challenges and opportunities demand unique solutions. Transplanting knowledge structure, formations, and practices developed and employed in tertiary care and specialist facilities results in a lack of goodness of fit. Context and local knowledge are critical to the understanding of illness in primary care. Universal abstractions may not fit local reality and artificially forced structures. Primary care should be able to choose a different framework for the management of psychiatric and emotional problems. Contexts can not only change medical practice but should also be able to change medical perspectives.

The complexity of the issues related to the diagnosis and management of such presentations demands a re-evaluation of the issues. The suggested approaches are rooted in primary care, have been found to be useful, and can be successfully employed within busy surgical and medical clinics.

4 The Conceptual Basis of the Approach to Managing Psychiatric Disorders in General Hospital Settings

The conceptual approach to recognizing psychiatric presentations in general medical settings includes the identification of the clinical presentation and exclusion of medical and organic causes. The steps in management are: treating medical causes when identified, and the symptomatic management of the clinical presentation.

INTRODUCTION

The approach to psychiatric disorders recommended in this book is based on many years of working in primary care and general hospital settings. With this came the recognition that specialist psychiatric perspectives are inappropriate for such situations. The milder, mixed, and less-than-typical clinical presentations seen demanded the need to empower physicians using more relevant medical perspectives rather than inundate them with psychiatric jargon and specialist perceptions, which tend to disempower.

The experience of working in general hospital facilities also highlighted the unsuitability of the many available psychiatric protocols, with their time-consuming details. The need to tailor management strategies to the available time in busy general hospital settings also played a major part in the development of these simple protocols, using a single and simple overarching framework. This brief framework is the abstraction of what competent clinicians actually do when faced with psychiatric presentations in busy medical settings. Their brevity, while sharply contrasting with the complex protocols used by psychiatrists and transplanted to primary care, employs sound conceptual principles of management employed in medicine across settings.

CONCEPTUAL BASIS OF PSYCHIATRIC DIAGNOSIS AND TREATMENT

The current inability to identify specific biological abnormalities and the consequent absence of laboratory markers to diagnose psychiatric disorders has meant a sole reliance on clinical manifestations of mental illness for diagnosis. Consequently, the basis of diagnosis in psychiatry is the recognition of constellations of symptoms and signs, i.e. syndrome. The syndromic nature of psychiatric diagnosis automatically implies heterogeneous causation. The diverse causes argue for the need to identify specific etiology, if present, especially the medical and neurological causes that produce psychiatric syndromes. The identification of particular causes mandates specific and targeted treatment strategies. In addition to the management of the causes identified, the syndrome will also require symptomatic treatment to relieve symptoms. Syndromes for which no medical causes are identified require symptomatic treatment.

In summary, the steps in psychiatric diagnosis are:

• Identify specific syndrome
• Rule out medical causes.

The steps in management are:

• Treat medical causes, if identified
• Treat symptomatically.

For example, in patients presenting with symptoms of depression, the clinician has to document the presence of the full syndrome/constellation of depression. He/she will then have to proceed to rule out medical, neurological, and endocrine causes of depression. Common medical causes include tumors of the brain, hypothyroidism, and diabetes mellitus. When such specific causes are identified, they will have to be treated using particular treatments. In addition, these patients will require antidepressant medication to relieve them of their distressing symptoms.

Similar steps are required for the management of psychosis. The syndrome of psychosis is identified on the basis of the constellation of symptoms, including strange beliefs (delusions), hearing voices/seeing visions (hallucinations), and grossly abnormal behavior. Once the syndrome is recognized, medical and organic causes will have to be excluded. If medical causes are identified (e.g. temporal lobe epilepsy or hyperthyroidism), then they have to be specifically treated. In addition, antipsychotic medication will be required to control the psychotic symptoms. In patients in whom no medical causes are identified, the management is essentially symptomatic.

SUB-CATEGORIZATION IN TERTIARY CARE: INTENT AND CONSEQUENCES

Psychiatric classification was based on two premises: (i) symptom counts improve reliability of diagnosis and (ii) sub-categorization of broad categories will result in homogeneous grouping, facilitating the elicitation of biological etiology. The focus on reliability mandated the need to employ objective symptoms and minimize clinician interpretation. Consequently, the evaluation of context, which involved subject assessment, was discounted. The hope that sub-categorization will result in homogeneous categories has recently been abandoned, recognizing the futility of the approach. Current psychiatric diagnostic heads, despite the phenomenal increase in their number, stubbornly remain heterogeneous on symptoms, disability, functioning, treatment response, course, and outcome. Variations within diagnostic heads are as great as those between categories.

Consequently, psychiatry currently emphasizes the need to tailor treatment options and individualize management strategies based on particular symptoms, specific disability, detailed assessment of functioning, and livelihood issues. In essence, despite its elaborate assessment schedules, complex classificatory system, and specific treatment protocols, psychiatry also approaches clinical presentations by identifying broad grouping and individualizes patient management by symptomatically treating individuals.

PROBLEMS WITH USING SPECIALIST APPROACHES IN GENERAL HOSPITALS

The specialist approach pursued by psychiatrists may be useful in tertiary and specialist facilities, where the referral system channels severe, complex, and classical cases for expert care. However, it is much less useful when transplanted to primary care and general hospital settings, where the reality is very different. Nevertheless, many training programs in psychiatry for general physicians use specialist perspectives and protocols. Most programs transfer knowledge and rarely attempt to focus on the necessary skills required to manage such disorders. The failure of general physicians to actually use these specialist approaches when they return to primary care results in a lack of confidence, making them wary of psychiatric presentations and, consequently, such patients. Most prefer to refer such patients for specialist attention rather than attempt to manage them. Nevertheless, such patients referred for professional care tend not to go to psychiatric facilities or see psychiatrists, as mental disorders continue to be stigmatizing. They tend to shop for treatment within general medical facilities and the vicious cycle of the lack of care and shopping continues.

THE IDENTIFICATION OF BROAD SYNDROMES

The first step in managing psychiatric presentations is the recognition of the clinical presentation. Psychiatric diagnoses are syndromes, implying that they are collections of signs and symptoms. Their syndrome status implies their heterogeneity in terms of etiology, clinical features, treatment response, course, and outcome. Traditionally, psychiatry has also identified sub-syndromes within these broad syndromes. While these sub-syndromes are useful in tertiary psychiatric facilities, they have limited use in primary care, where patients present with milder and mixed clinical presentations. For example, symptoms of anxiety and symptoms of depression are commonly seen in the same patient in primary care, making differentiation into classical and distinct syndromes very difficult. In addition, the use of symptomatic rather than syndrome-specific treatments in psychiatry argues for managing the broad syndrome/general clinical presentation.

THE BROAD SYNDROMES AND PRESENTATIONS USEFUL IN GENERAL HOSPITALS

The broad syndromes and clinical presentations considered necessary and useful in general hospital settings include the following:

- *Delirium* – acute confusion and disorientation
- *Dementia* – chronic memory and severe cognitive dysfunction
- *Substance Use and Dependence*
- *Psychosis* – strange beliefs, hallucinations and grossly abnormal behavior
- *Somatic Symptoms*

These clinical presentations are discussed using a single framework. The principles are similar to those used in psychiatry and tertiary care, the difference being that broad clinical presentations commonly seen in general hospitals are highlighted instead of specific syndromes.

THE DEVELOPMENT OF A SINGLE PROTOCOL

The 10-step general protocol has been developed over the last decade. The protocols initially started as simple teaching modules for the common psychiatric presentations seen in primary care. The first module developed was for the management of medically unexplained symptoms. The many years of informal testing in primary care and its use for teaching physicians and medical students allowed for its refinement. Its success in the field and the feedback of the many physicians who have employed it gave the authors the confidence to pursue the simplification of protocols for other common psychiatric disorders. The use of these simple protocols for many years and the realization of the difficulty in remembering minor variations for the management of each of these conditions resulted in its synthesis into the currently formulated single general protocol. This approach attempts to synthesize the many chapters into a single protocol to present a clear and concise approach to management in primary care. Its use will allow for repeated practice, which will transfer the necessary skills, increase the physician's confidence, and provide a sense of mastery and satisfaction, reinforcing the management of psychiatric presentations.

Section II

Common Clinical Presentations in Adults

5 Delirium

The clinical presentation of delirium is characterized by difficulties with attention and concentration, and disorientation to time, place, and person. Additional symptoms of restlessness, delusions, hallucinations, abnormal behavior, and sleep disturbance can color the picture. Delirium is commonly seen in the elderly, in patients admitted to the intensive care unit, and during the postoperative period.

As all causes of delirium are medical, neurological, or endocrine abnormalities, they will have to be excluded by physical examination and laboratory investigations. The medical basis of the condition needs to be treated. Agitation and sleep disturbance are managed using small doses of antipsychotic medication. Reorienting the patient to time, place, and person is part of essential management.

INTRODUCTION

A common psychiatric presentation among hospitalized patients in a general medical and surgical setting is delirium. Delirium or acute confusional state is a transient global disorder of cognition. It is more common among the hospitalized, the frail and elderly, postoperative patients, those admitted to intensive care units, and those with compromised mental state (e.g. dementia). The condition is a medical emergency associated with increased morbidity and mortality rates. This chapter discusses the recognition and management of delirium.

WHAT IS THE CLINICAL PICTURE IN DELIRIUM?

Delirium is characterized by a rapid onset and fluctuating course of clouding of consciousness, attention deficits, cognitive disturbances, psychomotor changes, and sleep disturbance. Reduced ability to direct, focus, sustain, and shift attention is common. Reduced orientation to the environment is the classical presentation. The disturbance develops over a short period (hours or days) and represents a change from baseline attention and awareness. Disturbances in cognition including memory deficits, disorientation, and difficulty in language, visuospatial ability, and perception, may be additional symptoms. The disturbance should not be part of an evolving neurocognitive condition with severely reduced levels of arousal such as coma.

WHAT IS THE PREVALENCE OF DELIRIUM?

It is commonly seen among the hospitalized, the elderly, postoperative patients, those admitted to intensive care units, and those with compromised mental state, e.g. dementia. The overall prevalence of delirium in the community is low (1%–2%). The estimated prevalence of delirium in patients presenting to emergency departments (15%–25%), among postoperative patients (25%–50%), and those in intensive and critical care units (70%–90%) is much higher. Delirium may be increased in the context of functional impairment, impaired mobility, a history of falls, low levels of activity, and the use of drugs and medication, particularly alcohol and anticholinergics.

What is the recognition rate of delirium?

Many studies have documented that physicians do not identify a majority of patients with delirium.

What happens to patients who do not get help from physicians?

The causes of delirium are always medical and neurological. The majority of individuals recover with or without specific treatment. However, early recognition and intervention reduces the period of hospitalization, while the failure to recognize such dysfunction results in the prolongation of illness and longer hospital stays. In addition, the mortality rates of patients with delirium are much higher than those who are not delirious. Delirium may progress to stupor, coma, seizures, or death, particularly if the underlying causes remain untreated. The recognition of delirium and the treatment of the underlying medical cause(s) improve medical outcomes and contribute to good medical practice.

What are the different clinical presentations of delirium?

Generally, two patterns of delirium are recognized: (i) delirium with agitation (hyperactive) and (ii) quiet delirium (hypoactive). The former is often identified as the patient is disturbed and disrupts the routine care in the hospital or intensive care unit. The latter is often missed as the patient is not disruptive and physicians do not attempt to routinely test people to check for delirium. Hyperactive delirium is more common with medication side-effects and drug withdrawal, while hypoactive states are usually seen in older people.

Will I be able to make a clinical diagnosis of delirium?

The diagnosis of delirium is based on the recognition of the clinical syndrome. Recognizing delirium is not difficult in clinical practice and can be done based on a detailed history from relatives and observations from hospital and intensive care staff.

What are the clinical features of delirium?

Delirium manifests clinically with a wide range of neuropsychiatric abnormalities. The clinical hallmarks are decreased attention span and a waxing and waning type of confusion. The major symptoms include clouding and fluctuation of consciousness, difficulties in attention, and disorientation to time, place, and person. Visual and auditory hallucinations and paranoid delusions may also be present. The patient may have associated neurological symptoms, such as dysarthria, dysphasia, tremor, and asterixis. The disturbance is usually characterized by an acute onset of symptoms, over hours or days, and may fluctuate in severity from hour to hour with a worsening state, particularly at night.

Disturbance in the sleep–wake cycle including daytime sleepiness, nighttime agitation, difficulty in falling asleep, and excessive sleepiness throughout the day and wakefulness throughout the night are additional features that support a diagnosis of delirium. Delirium can also be superimposed on a dementia. Attenuated delirium syndrome that does not meet full syndrome suggests milder or early presentation.

WHAT ARE THE CAUSES OF DELIRIUM?

Common reversible causes of delirium include hypoxia, hypoglycemia, hyperthermia, anticholinergic medication, and alcohol or sedative withdrawal. Sudden withdrawal of substances (e.g. alcohol and opioids) and medication withdrawal (e.g. sedative, hypnotic, and anxiolytic), particularly during periods of hospitalization, should be ruled out.

The others include infections, metabolic abnormalities, structural lesions of the brain, postoperative states, sensory or sleep deprivation, fecal impaction, urinary retention, and change of environment. Often, particularly in the critically ill and in elderly hospitalized patients, delirium may have multiple etiologies. Occasionally, no clear etiology is immediately apparent. Delirium in children is often associated with febrile illness, seizures, and medication (e.g. anticholinergics).

ARE THERE LABORATORY TESTS FOR DELIRIUM?

While there is a generalized slowing on electroencephalography (EEG) and occasional fast activity, EEG is insufficiently sensitive and specific for diagnostic use. The diagnosis is clinical, and the identification of laboratory pathology indicative of the underlying medical and neurological condition is enough to make a definitive diagnosis.

WILL I BE ABLE TO DIAGNOSE THE CAUSE OF DELIRIUM?

The identification of a specific cause for the clinical presentation of delirium is based on a detailed history, physical examination, and laboratory investigations. Acute onset of the confusion, its short duration, and fluctuating course, with worsening at night, are diagnostic. A detailed mental status examination, which checks for orientation to time, place, and person, is crucial. Attention deficits, confusion, visual and auditory hallucinations, fear, and perplexity are also pointers to a diagnosis of delirium.

A physical examination (e.g. high blood pressure and pulse rate, rapid respiration, signs of consolidation, and signs of stroke) and appropriate laboratory tests (e.g. complete blood count, serum creatinine, blood sugar, serum electrolyte, urine protein and microscopy, thyroid stimulating hormone, and CT scan) will be necessary to identify the specific cause.

WILL A SINGLE PROTOCOL HELP IN THE MANAGEMENT OF DIFFERENT TYPES OF PATIENTS?

Yes. The protocol contains all the essential steps in the management of these conditions.

BOX 5.1   QUIET DELIRIUM

A 70-year-old man was brought to the Emergency Department with a one-week history of fever and loss of appetite. His relatives noticed that he was not aware of his surroundings and was confused. His personal care had deteriorated. His sleep was disturbed. On examination, he was disorientated to time, place, and person. Physical examination and laboratory investigations suggested pneumonia.

He was started on antibiotics. A very small dose of haloperidol (0.25 mg at bedtime) was given. He recovered his mental functions with treatment.

BOX 5.2   AGITATED DELIRIUM

A 75-year-old woman was brought to Emergency Department with a two-day history of confusion and an inability to recognize relatives. She was restless and agitated. Physical examination did not reveal any abnormality. However, urine microscopy showed a high white blood cell count, suggesting a urinary tract infection.

She was started on antibiotics. Tab. risperidone, 0.25 mg twice a day, was added to control her restlessness. The dose was increased to 1 mg in divided doses. She settled down in a few days and recovered her original level of function.

BOX 5.3   DELIRIUM IN A PATIENT WITH DEMENTIA

An 80-year-old man was brought to the emergency department with a two-day history of marked restlessness and agitation. He also has a one-year history of significant decline in memory, inability to dress, poor personal care, and difficulty with shopping. He was diagnosed to have dementia and was started on acetylcholine esterase inhibitors. His recent change in behavior was distressing to his family. A detailed assessment of his mental state suggested significant disorientation. He was not able to recognize his relatives and was not aware of the surroundings. This was in contrast to his previous state where he related well with his relatives and was able to look after his personal needs despite failing memory. Although he did not complain of dysuria or increased urinary frequency, his urine microscopy documented increased cell counts and his urine culture grew *Escherichia coli*.

He was treated with small doses of risperidone to control his agitation. His cognitive state improved with a course of antibiotics and he returned to his previous level of functioning.

> **BOX 5.4   DELIRIUM DURING ELECTIVE SURGERY**
>
> A 50-year-old woman was admitted to hospital for an elective hysterectomy for dysfunctional uterine bleeding. Her preoperative investigations were normal and she had an uneventful surgery. However, she reported sleep disturbance, tremor, and restlessness during the immediate postoperative period. Her attention was impaired and she occasionally misidentified the hospital staff.
>
> A detailed history revealed chronic use of alcohol in a dependence pattern. She had not revealed her substance use to her gynecologist. She improved with substitution with benzodiazepines and with injectable thiamine.

> **BOX 5.5   ENVIRONMENTAL INTERVENTIONS FOR DELIRIUM**
>
> - Adequate daytime lighting and diminished nighttime lighting to simulate day–night cycle
> - Regular attempts at orienting patient with calendars and clocks
> - Detailed and clear introductions of new people and procedures
> - Providing the right amount of stimulation for the patient; avoiding over-stimulation, recognizing under-stimulation and intervening
> - Providing hearing aids, spectacles to correct sensory deficits
> - Encouraging sleep
> - Maintaining safety
> - Regular interaction to achieve familiarity and consistency for patient
> - Having family members stay is helpful; bringing personal effects from home is useful

WHAT ARE THE TEN STEPS?

The ten steps in management are:

1. Recognize the clinical presentation
2. Acknowledge distress
3. Elicit the patient's and the family's perspective
4. Take a focused history; carry out physical examination and laboratory investigations to rule out medical problems
5. Educate the patients, their families, and hospital staff about the nature of illness and its treatment
6. Prescribe medication
7. Discuss the role of stress as cause and consequence of illness
8. Elaborate coping strategies
9. Negotiate a treatment plan, compliance, participation, and responsibility
10. Give an appointment for review.

Step 1. Recognize the clinical presentation of delirium

Eliciting a history of disorientation to time, place, and person can easily identify delirium. Mild disorientation results in the lack of appreciation of time, while marked disorientation results in an inability to recognize people and the place. Other important features of delirium include a decreased attention span, and a waxing and waning type of confusion. There is clouding and fluctuation of consciousness.

The patient could be either restless and agitated or withdrawn. Visual and auditory hallucinations and fleeting paranoid delusions may also be present. The patient may have associated neurological symptoms such as dysarthria, dysphasia, tremor, and asterixis.

The disturbance is classically characterized by an acute onset of symptoms, over hours or days. The disturbance may fluctuate in severity from hour to hour, with a worsening state, particularly at night. A detailed history and clinical examination are necessary to establish the clinical presentation.

Psychosis (characterized by strange beliefs, hallucinations, grossly abnormal behavior), which is not associated with clouding of consciousness and disorientation, will need to be excluded.

Step 2. Acknowledge distress

The sudden onset of disturbance places a heavy burden on caregivers, family members, and the hospital staff. Acknowledging the distress to caregivers caused by delirium is mandatory.

Step 3. Elicit the patient's and the family's perspective on symptoms

Providing appropriate reassurance is an important part of the medical consultation. It is most effective if based on the patient's actual concerns. Asking patients, relatives, and the hospital staff what they think or fear is wrong with the patient is useful in addressing specific concerns. (The relatives often report: "He has been very restless, abusive, and he even hit me" or "He constantly accuses me of stealing his possessions".)

Many of the beliefs held by the family and hospital staff may contradict the biomedical model of the illness. They may consider violence and disinhibited behavior as a deliberate provocation rather than consider it as part of a disease process. The beliefs held by the family and the hospital staff need to be discussed for presenting alternative biomedical explanations.

Step 4. Take a focused history; carry out physical examination and laboratory investigations

Delirium must be distinguished from a psychotic disorder, which is not generally associated with confusion or a change in the level of consciousness. The acuteness of onset, fluctuating severity, and disturbance of consciousness of delirium is helpful in distinguishing it from dementia, in which the patient is generally alert, the onset is usually gradual and does not fluctuate.

The establishing of deficits in attention and concentration, the disorientation to time, place, and person, and the clouding of consciousness of acute onset and short duration clinches the diagnosis. The next step will be the identification of the medical cause, which has contributed to the delirium.

Physical examination should be carried out to exclude high or very low blood pressure, dehydration, jaundice, cyanosis, fever, localizing signs of infection, signs of meningeal irritation, papilledema, pneumonia, etc.

The common laboratory tests which may need to be done to establish causation include: complete blood count, electrolytes, blood glucose, renal and liver function tests, and urine analysis for proteinuria and white cells. Neuroimaging, EEG, ECG, and pulse oxymetry are also useful.

A brief yet systematic examination will go a long way in identifying specific causes of delirium. The extent of laboratory investigation, which should be done, is dependent on the clinical presentation and the patient's socioeconomic status. Basic tests may be required to identify conditions, which do not have clinical signs and pathognemonic manifestations.

Step 5. Educate the patient about the illness and treatment

The disturbed behavior or complete apathy due to delirium and the clouding of consciousness are distressing both for the family and the hospital staff. Educating the family and caregivers about the disease status is mandatory. It becomes necessary to address the family's and attending health professional's beliefs and misconceptions about the condition. Discussing the nature of the condition, the need to manage causal and risk factors, and the role of medication and psychosocial treatments is necessary.

Vital functions (e.g. heart rate, blood pressure, respiration, temperature, intake, and output) should be regularly monitored. Fluid and nutrition should be managed. The patient's medications should be carefully reviewed; non-essential medication should be discontinued, and doses of needed medication should be kept as low as possible. Severely delirious patients who are agitated and wandering benefit from constant observation and reassurance, which may help avoid the use of physical restraints. Reorientation techniques, such as the use of calendars, clocks, and family photos, may be helpful. The environment should be stable, quiet, and well lit. Support from a familiar nurse and the family should be encouraged. Sensory deficits should be corrected with eyeglasses and hearing aids.

Step 6. Prescribe medication

Treating the specifically identified causes of delirium and risk factors is necessary. The control of hypertension and diabetes mellitus, the treatment of infections (respiratory, urinary tract, and central nervous system), the correction of dehydration and electrolyte imbalance, or the management of liver and kidney decompensation, when contributory to the delirium, is mandatory. Substance use will need to be managed. Medication for physical conditions, which is deemed to be not absolutely necessary, should be withdrawn.

Antipsychotics are the medication of choice in delirium. Older neuroleptics such as haloperidol are useful, but have adverse neurological effects. Newer neuroleptics, such as risperidone, olanzapine, and quetiapine, relieve the symptoms while minimizing the adverse effects. Smaller doses than used in functional psychosis are required (e.g. 0.25–1 mg/day of haloperidol; 0.5–1 mg/day of risperidone; 2.5–5 mg/day of olanzapine; 25–100 mg/day of quetiapine).

Benzodiazepines are reserved for delirium resulting from seizures (e.g. 1–3 mg lorazepam/day), withdrawal from alcohol/sedative hypnotics (e.g. 2–8 mg lorazepam/day), or when unknown substances may have been ingested. They must be used cautiously as they can cause respiratory depression, especially in patients who are elderly or debilitated. Benzodiazepines are best avoided as they are addictive and could cause a paradoxical worsening of symptoms, especially in the elderly. Anticholinergic medication is also contraindicated as it may worsen the memory impairment and increase the confusion.

An attempt should be made to taper the medication once the symptoms are under control. The principles in medication management in older people include starting at lower doses with much slower increases in dose. This is also necessary in patients with liver and kidney disease or dysfunction.

Step 7. Discuss the role of stress especially on relatives and hospital staff

The burden of delirium on the family members and hospital staff should be discussed. Educate the family regarding the etiology and course of the problem. Providing reassurance that delirium often is temporary and is the result of a medical condition may be beneficial to both patients and their families. Suggest that family members or friends visit the patient, ideally one at a time, and provide a calm and structured environment. Psychological support will be required for relatives.

Step 8. Elaborate coping strategies

Providing a calm atmosphere is necessary. The use of physical restraints may be necessary for a short duration to prevent the patient from harming himself, especially if he is not cooperative with the medical management of his underlying disease. Adequate lighting, daily attempts at orientation of the patient, and the use of large calendars and clocks are helpful. Unfamiliar people should be introduced and hospital and laboratory procedures explained.

Step 9. Negotiate a treatment plan

Most patients with delirium recover with adequate treatment. The identification of the underlying medical cause may require further investigation and stay in the hospital/intensive care. The course in hospital and the investigations and treatment need to be negotiated with the family.

Step 10. Give a specific appointment for review

Regular and daily review of the clinical status is required. Psychotropic medication can be gradually tapered after the mental status improves. A regular review of the patient's condition is mandatory for fine-tuning medication and for providing support and advice to relatives. The antipsychotic medication can be tapered and withdrawn in about 3 months.

WILL I BE ABLE TO CURE THE PATIENT'S DISEASE?

The treatment of delirium usually results in good outcomes and cure in the majority of patients. Early diagnosis and appropriate management of the cause are mandatory.

WHEN SHOULD I REFER A PATIENT FOR SPECIALIST HELP?

Many patients with delirium settle with the treatment of the underlying cause, antipsychotic medication, and supportive measures. However, psychiatric consultation may be indicated for the management of behavioral problems, such as severe agitation or aggressive behavior.

CONCLUSION

The recognition of delirium is crucial to managing patients in an in-patient hospital setting. Identifying specific causes and risk factors and their management are mandatory.

6 Dementia

Dementia is characterized by multiple cognitive dysfunctions, including deterioration in complex attention, executive function, learning and memory, language, perceptual-motor function, and social cognition. The symptoms are usually gradual in onset and progressive, and result in impairment in social and occupational function. Dementia is commonly seen in older people.

The identification of the medical and neurological cause of the condition, the exclusion of reversible causes of dementia, and the control of risk factors, such as diabetes mellitus, hypertension, hypercholesterolemia, smoking, and the excessive use of alcohol, are mandatory.

The mainstay of treatment is the psychosocial management of the condition. Acetylcholine esterase inhibitors cannot cure the disease, but can delay its progress. Patients with psychotic symptoms, and depression and anxiety will require small doses of antipsychotic and antidepressant medication, respectively.

INTRODUCTION

The increase in longevity of the population has resulted in an increase in the number of older people in society. Illness among the elderly has a significant impact on their quality of life and on the burden of disease. Dementia, now called major neurocognitive disorder, is one of the most significant contributors to the burden of disease. The condition is a cause of severe disability and, consequently, burden.

A significant proportion of the elderly population, especially those attending hospital facilities, report subjective memory loss. This chapter discusses a simple approach to managing such patients in primary care and general medical settings.

WHAT ARE THE COMMON PSYCHIATRIC AND PSYCHOSOCIAL PROBLEMS SEEN IN OLDER PEOPLE ATTENDING PRIMARY CARE AND GENERAL HOSPITALS?

Subjective memory loss and impaired cognitive function are common presenting complaints among older people. However, the general population expects such memory impairment and cognitive decline as part of the normal process of aging. The possibility of a disease state contributing to such memory complaints is a recent concept.

WHAT IS THE PREVALENCE OF DEMENTIA?

The prevalence varies by age and etiological subtype. It increases with age, and estimates of 1%–2% have been reported in people over 65 years with figures reaching up to 30% over 85 years of age.

How common are memory complaints in primary care?

The majority of the elderly who visit hospital report some form of memory and cognitive impairment. The severity and quality differs, and requires a detailed assessment to exclude disease states.

What happens to patients who do not get help from physicians?

The inability of physicians to identify disease causes of memory dysfunction, its acceptance as part of normal ageing, and a lack of skill in managing such presentations often results in the physician downplaying the importance of the condition and ignoring patient distress. The lack of recognition of dementia and related memory problems leads to continued suffering and impaired quality of life for the elderly.

What are the different types of memory dysfunction among the elderly?

Generally, three patterns of memory impairment can be recognized: (i) age-related cognitive decline; (ii) mild cognitive impairment (now referred to as minor neurocognitive disorder); and (iii) dementia. The need to identify the specific pattern of dysfunction and disease is cardinal to good management.

What are the major cognitive domains?

Cognition is now divided into the following domains: complex attention, executive function, learning and memory, language, perceptual-motor function, and social cognition.

What are the examples of cognitive dysfunction?

The examples of cognitive dysfunction are given in Table 6.1.

How can I differentiate dementia from normal age-related memory problems?

While aging is often associated with some reduction in cognitive abilities, these are significantly impaired in dementia. Such dysfunction progresses along a continuum and is dimensional with age-related decline at one end and dementia on the other. The stage of intermediate dysfunction is called mild cognitive impairment. A simple way to distinguish the three conditions is given in Table 6.2.

Dementia is differentiated from normal aging and mild cognitive impairment by the presence of multiple cognitive impairments. The presence of any of these additional cognitive impairments is sufficient to make a diagnosis of dementia. These symptoms should cause social and occupational impairment, should be of at least 6 months' duration, and should be progressive. People with milder impairment can cope with minimal help from caregivers; those with dementia require significant support for functioning.

TABLE 6.1

Examples of Cognitive Dysfunction

Cognitive domain	Examples of problems
Complex attention	1. Easily distracted by competing events in the environments (e.g. inability to hold a conversation when watching television or listening to the radio) 2. Inability to recall recent conversation or new information 3. Inability to perform mental calculations
Executive function	1. Unable to focus on more than one task at a time; unable to resume task, if interrupted 2. Inability to make plans and execute them 3. Problems in decision making and requiring help from others
Learning and memory	1. Problems in immediate and recent memory; repeats information, often within same conversation, unable to remember short lists of items 2. Semantic and autobiographical memory impaired later in course of illness
Language	1. Naming and word finding difficulty; prefers general pronouns to names; difficulty in recalling names 2. Reduction in fluency of language and spontaneity of speech output; grammatical errors 3. Difficulty in comprehending language and commands; Difficulty in understanding and following simple conversations; the decreased ability to read and understand newspaper/news in the presence of reasonable vision, speech and hearing
Perceptual-motor	1. Difficulty in using familiar tools; driving motor vehicle 2. Difficulty in navigating familiar environments 3. Difficulty in identifying common objects 4. Difficulty to wear clothes correctly 5. Inability to perform activities related to personal grooming (e.g. comb hair and brush teeth)
Social cognition	1. Insensitivity to social standards of dress and conversation 2. Makes decisions without regard to personal safety 3. Lacks insight into behavior

CAN DEMENTIA BE COLORED BY OTHER PSYCHIATRIC PRESENTATIONS?

Yes. Many different psychiatric symptoms can be concurrently present along with deterioration in cognitive function. In fact, some of these symptoms may be so prominent that they can mask the clinical picture of dementia.

Psychotic symptoms can be present, particularly paranoid delusions (belief that other people plan to harm, persecute, or steal), referential beliefs (that other people are talking about them), and auditory and visual hallucinations. These symptoms can be associated with significant insomnia, loss of appetite, and weight loss. They can

TABLE 6.2

Characteristics to Distinguish Different Forms of Dementia

Characteristic	Age-related memory impairment	Mild cognitive impairment	Dementia
Evidence of progressive cognitive impairment of 6 months' duration from history and clinical examination	Present	Present	Present
Associated social and occupational dysfunction	Absent	Present	Present
Presence of significant dysfunction in cognitive domains with impairments in multiple areas	Absent	Absent	Present

also result in preoccupation, social withdrawal, and social isolation. Increased talk, expansive ideas, irritability, anger, and abusive and assaultive behavior can also color the picture.

Depressive symptoms, sadness, crying, worry, loneliness, and suicidal ideation can be associated with significant insomnia, loss of appetite, and reduction in weight. Others can present with anxiety and increased use of alcohol, sedatives, hypnotics, and anxiolytics.

All older people presenting with psychiatric symptoms should be evaluated in detail for excluding concomitant delirium and dementia as their probability is much higher at extremes of age. All subtypes of dementia have a high risk of being associated with psychotic, depressive, or anxiety symptoms. While psychiatric syndromes will necessarily have to be treated symptomatically, the recognition of cognitive disorders is crucial for long-term management and care.

WILL I BE ABLE TO MAKE A CLINICAL DIAGNOSIS OF DEMENTIA?

Yes, you will be able to diagnose dementia. The diagnosis of dementia is based on the recognition of the clinical syndrome. Differentiating dementia from normal aging, normal age-related memory impairment, and mild cognitive impairment is not difficult in clinical practice and can be done based on a detailed history from relatives. While formal diagnosis of dementia requires detailed psychometric evaluation, provisional diagnosis can be reached through reports from caregivers and by direct observation.

WHAT ARE THE CAUSES OF DEMENTIA?

Dementia is a syndrome caused by diverse diseases of the brain including cerebrovascular disease, tumors, chronic infections (HIV, syphilis, Prion disease), degenerative diseases (Alzheimer, fronto-temporal degeneration, Lewy body disease, Parkinson, Huntington), subdural hematoma, traumatic brain injury and normal pressure hydrocephalus.

The risk for dementia increases with the following systemic diseases: hypertension, diabetes, hypothyroidism, vitamin deficiencies (B12, folic acid, and niacin), and hypercholesterolemia. Cognitive dysfunction can also be due to substance dependence. They can also have multiple etiologies.

WHAT ARE THE GENERAL RISK FACTORS FOR DEMENTIA?

High blood pressure, uncontrolled diabetes mellitus, and dyslipidemia increase the risk of developing the condition and need to be managed with appropriate medication. Possible nutritional deficiencies will need vitamin supplementation. Substance abuse adds to the probability of cognitive decline.

WILL I BE ABLE TO DIAGNOSE THE CAUSE OF DEMENTIA?

The identification of a specific cause for the clinical presentation of dementia is based on a detailed history, physical examination, and laboratory investigations. A physical examination and appropriate laboratory tests (e.g. complete blood count, serum creatinine, blood sugar levels, lipids, vitamin levels, thyroid stimulating hormone, and CT scan) will be necessary to identify the specific cause and exclude treatable causes of dementia. High blood pressure, thyroid swelling, delayed/absent ankle jerk, and skin manifestations of vitamin deficiencies must be excluded.

WHAT IS THE COURSE OF DEMENTIA?

The course of the condition varies according to subtype. While some subtypes are static (e.g. due to traumatic brain injury), others progress over time (e.g. cerebral degenerative diseases such as Alzheimer and fronto-temporal dementias). Fluctuations in course may be worsened by episodes of superimposed delirium.

WILL A SINGLE PROTOCOL HELP IN THE MANAGEMENT OF DIFFERENT TYPES OF PATIENTS WITH DEMENTIA?

Yes. The protocol contains all the essential steps in the management of this condition.

WHAT IS THE BASIS OF THE SUGGESTED PROTOCOL?

The approach described is based on the use of both pharmacological and psychosocial treatments for the condition. The steps, the sequence and their rationale are briefly described.

WHAT ARE THE TEN STEPS?

The ten steps in management are:

1. Recognize the clinical presentation
2. Acknowledge distress
3. Elicit the patient's and the family's perspective
4. Take a focused history, and carry out physical examination and laboratory investigations to rule out medical problems
5. Educate the patient about the nature of illness and its treatment

6. Prescribe medication
7. Discuss the role of stress as cause and consequence of illness
8. Elaborate coping strategies
9. Negotiate a treatment plan, compliance, participation, and responsibility
10. Give an appointment for review.

Step 1. Recognize the clinical presentation of dementia

Diagnosing dementia involves the elicitation of a history of progressive decline in multiple cognitive domains: complex attention, executive function, learning and memory, language, perceptual-motor function, and social cognition. The decline results in social and occupational impairment and is progressive.

Dementia should be differentiated from normal age-related cognitive decline and mild cognitive impairment by the presence of impairments in multiple domains of cognitive functions, severity of deterioration, progression over time, loss of independence in functioning, and amount of help required from caregivers.

Dementia can also be associated with the following symptoms: restlessness, wandering, disinhibited behavior, depressive symptoms, incontinence, anger, irritability, abusive or assaultive behavior, and sleep disturbance. Psychotic symptoms, depression, and anxiety are also common. These have to be enquired into as they are very distressing to relatives, increase the burden of disease on the family, and can be managed with treatment.

Other common clinical presentations, which can co-occur and need to be identified and treated are:

*   delirium with acute confusion and disorientation to time, place, and person
*   psychosis with strange beliefs, hallucinations, and grossly abnormal behavior
*   severe depression with crying episodes, sleep disturbance, and suicidal ideation

Step 2. Acknowledge distress

The burden on caregivers and on family members is considerable and can result in depressive symptoms. Acknowledging the distress caused by dementia on the patient and particularly on the family is mandatory. It is often the women in the family (wife/daughter-in-law) who are the primary caregivers and bear the brunt of the disease. Acknowledging distress reflects an empathetic attitude, and contributes to establishing an effective rapport and the formation of a therapeutic alliance, which are essential in facilitating care and improvement.

Step 3. Elicit the patient's and the family's perspective on symptoms

Providing appropriate reassurance is an important part of the medical consultation. It is most effective if based on the patient's actual concerns. Discussing with patients and relatives what they think or fear is wrong is useful in addressing specific concerns (e.g. "It is part of normal aging" or "He constantly accuses me of stealing his possessions and poisoning his food").

Many beliefs held by the family about dementia contradict the biomedical model of the illness. They may hold strong beliefs that the memory and brain dysfunction are due to normal aging and may not seek help even for distressing and treatable behavioral and psychological symptoms of dementia (e.g. restlessness, wandering, anger, agitation, abusive and assaultive behavior, incontinence, sleep disturbance, and crying episodes).

They may also hold multiple beliefs about the condition, which incorporate supernatural causation (e.g. karma, sin, black magic, and punishment), or subscribe to local cultural views that poor diet and nutrition, excessive work, and poverty are causal.

The patient's and family's beliefs need to be discussed before presenting alternative biomedical explanations. A failure to elicit or outright rejection of the patient's beliefs about the illness early in the consultation often proves disastrous. Eliciting such explanations will also allow for specific reassurance.

Step 4. Take a focused history; carry out physical examination and laboratory investigations

Dementia, being a syndrome caused by diverse diseases of the brain and by systemic conditions, requires a detailed history, a physical examination, and laboratory investigations to identify specific causes. The specific causes identified will have to be treated/managed. Patients without specific causes are considered to have Alzheimer disease. However, the risk factors for dementia will have to be identified and managed in all patients (e.g. hypertension, diabetes mellitus, hypercholesterolemia, nutritional deficiencies, and hypothyroidism).

The following conditions will have to be excluded by history and physical examination:

- cerebrovascular disease – stroke, lacunar infarcts, transient ischemic attacks
- tumors – projectile vomiting, papilledema
- chronic infections – HIV, syphilis, tuberculosis
- degenerative diseases – tremor, rigidity, bradykinesia, chorea suggestive of Parkinson or Huntington disease
- subdural hematoma – history of fall, fracture, head injury
- normal pressure hydrocephalous – ataxia, confusion, incontinence
- The risk for dementia increases with the following systemic diseases: hypertension, diabetes, hypothyroidism, vitamin deficiencies (B12, folic acid, and niacin), and hypercholesterolemia.

A physical examination and appropriate laboratory tests (e.g. complete blood counts, ESR, creatinine, sugar, lipids, vitamin B12, folic acid, and niacin levels, TSH, and CT scan) will be necessary to exclude treatable causes of dementia.

This brief yet systematic examination will go a long way in identifying specific and treatable causes of dementia. The extent of laboratory investigation is dependent on the clinical presentation and the patient's socioeconomic status. Basic tests may be required to identify conditions that do not have clinical signs and pathognomonic manifestations.

Delirium (acute episodes of disorientation and confusion), if present, requires the recognition and treatment of medical causes such as urinary tract infections and pneumonia.

Step 5. Educate the patient about the illness and treatment

The disability and burden of dementia is huge. Educating the patients and especially the family and caregivers is mandatory. It becomes necessary to address the patient's and the family's beliefs and misconceptions about the condition.

Discussing the nature of the condition, the need to manage risk factors and the role of medication and psychosocial treatments is necessary. The fact that lifestyle modification and psychosocial interventions are the mainstay of treatment needs to be emphasized. The fact that medications only delay the progression of the disease and do not improve lost function should be mentioned. The usefulness of medication in improving the quality of life for both the patient and the family, without implying the possibility of cure, needs to be conveyed.

Step 6. Prescribe medication

The currently available medication helps in delaying the dementing process: Acetylcholine esterase inhibitors such as donepezil (starting dose 5 mg at bedtime; increase to 10 mg after one month) and rivastigmine (starting dose 1.5 mg twice a day; gradually increase to 6 mg per day) are useful for mild to moderate severity. Memantine can be added for moderate to severe dementia (starting dose 5 mg twice a day; can be gradually increased to 10 mg twice a day).

Treating the specifically identified causes of dementia and risk factors is mandatory. The control of hypertension, diabetes mellitus, and dyslipidemia is required in patients with a history of these factors and those with a history of cerebrovascular conditions. Antiretroviral medication, antibiotics and antituberculosis medication are necessary for chronic infections. Tumors and other degenerative conditions of the brain will require specific management. Substance use will need to be managed. Medication for physical conditions, which is deemed to be not absolutely necessary, should be withdrawn.

Hearing voices, persecutory beliefs, suspicious ideas, agitation, aggression, and wandering need to be managed with small doses of antipsychotic medication (e.g. haloperidol 0.25 twice a day; risperidone 0.5 mg twice a day). The sedative antipsychotic quetiapine is useful for patients with sleep disturbance, agitation, and psychosis (25–100 mg at bedtime). While many antipsychotics come with a black box warning of increased cardiovascular risk, they are useful in managing people with distressing psychotic presentations.

Depression (crying episodes, pervasive sadness) may require antidepressant medication. The choice of antidepressant medication is based on whether the patient has sleep disturbance or not. Sedative antidepressants should be used in such patients. These include tricyclics (e.g. dothiepin, imipramine; 25–100 mg/day) and mirtazapine (3.75–15 mg/day). Selective serotonin reuptake inhibitors (SSRIs) can be used in people with distress, depression, and persistent pain without sleep disturbance. Fluoxetine, sertraline, citalopram, and escitalopram are non-sedative and have fewer side-effects than the tricyclic agents.

Benzodiazepines are best avoided as they are addictive, cause a worsening of memory impairment, can produce paradoxical excitement, and increase the frequency of falls and fractures.

BOX 6.1   DEMENTIA

A 70-year-old man was brought with a one-year history of failing memory, inability to wear his clothes correctly, and a few episodes of wandering out of his house. These symptoms were gradually progressive and were interfering with his day-to-day functioning. On examination, he could not recognize common objects or his relatives. There was no history of hypertension or diabetes mellitus. His routine blood investigations were within normal limits. His CT scan showed evidence of cortical atrophy.

He was diagnosed to have dementia and was started on tab. donepezil, 5 mg at bedtime, which was increased to 10 mg after a month. The relatives were advised about the nature of illness and its treatment. They were educated about the importance of psychosocial management of the condition. While there was no recovery to his premorbid state, his condition was more manageable after the treatment was initiated.

BOX 6.2   DEMENTIA WITH DEPRESSION

A 75-year-old woman was brought with a one-year history of sadness, crying episodes, loss of appetite, and reduced interest in her surroundings. She mentioned that life was not worth living and talked about a wish to die. On inquiry, her relatives also mentioned failing memory and an inability to recognize her close relatives. These symptoms were gradually progressive and were interfering with her day-to-day functioning. On examination, she could not recognize common objects or remember important milestones in her life. There was a history of hypertension and diabetes mellitus, and the relatives reported a history of two transient ischemic attacks, with complete recovery of motor function. Her routine blood investigations were within normal limits. Her CT scan showed evidence of cortical atrophy.

She was diagnosed to have dementia with depression. She was started on tab. donepezil, 5 mg at bedtime, which was increased to 10 mg after a month. She was also started on tab. sertraline, 25 mg in the morning, and the dose was increased to 50 mg after a week. The relatives were advised about the nature of the illness and its treatment. They were educated about the importance of psychosocial management of the condition. While there was no recovery to her premorbid memory state, her depression lifted.

Dementia and its manifestations may include the presence of psychosis and depression as mentioned above and would mandate the use of antipsychotic or antidepressant medication in addition to the strategies for treating dementia. There may also be the additional complication of delirium, which will be manifested as acute and recent onset of disorientation and confusion. Good management would imply the

BOX 6.3 DEMENTIA WITH PSYCHOSIS

An 80-year-old man was brought with a one-year history of expressing suspicions about his relatives. He frequently accused them of stealing his possessions and poisoning his food. He had reduced appetite and disturbed sleep. There was also a history of failing memory. On examination, he had persecutory delusions. He could not recognize common objects and misidentified his relatives. There was no history of hypertension or diabetes mellitus. His routine blood investigations were within normal limits. His CT scan showed evidence of cortical atrophy.

He was diagnosed to have dementia with psychosis. He was started on tab. donepezil, 5 mg at bedtime, which was increased to 10 mg after a month. Antipsychotic medication quetiapine, 25 mg at bedtime, was added and this was gradually increased to 100 mg over 2 weeks. The relatives were advised about the nature of the illness and its treatment. They were educated about the importance of psychosocial management of the condition. While his memory did not improve, he stopped accusing his relatives of persecuting him.

BOX 6.4 AGE-RELATED COGNITIVE DECLINE

A 65-year-old man reported to hospital with complaints of memory problems. He reported that he would occasionally misplace household objects and fail to remember names of people, who used to be his acquaintances. He mentioned that he had lost his ability to remember items on his weekly shopping list, which were never a problem previously. He lived independently, looked after his personal needs, cooked and cleaned his house and managed his finances. He also had a reasonable social life. He said he preferred a routine for his life and was coping well. He resorted to maintaining detailed diaries and appointment schedules. He always went to the market with a shopping list. He said that while his daughter did visit him every week, he did not depend on her or his friends for managing his life. However, he was worried that he may have dementia.

A detailed examination did not reveal major difficulties in complex attention, new learning, language, social cognition, perceptual-motor and executive function. He was reassured about his cognitive status. The use of daily routines and memory aides were reiterated. He was advised an annual review of his cognitive function and physical health.

recognition of such delirium, the identification of its causes, its management, and the provision of symptomatic relief with a small dose of antipsychotics.

Medication management in older people should start at lower doses, with much slower increases in dose. This is particularly necessary in patients with liver and kidney disease and dysfunction.

BOX 6.5   MILD COGNITIVE IMPAIRMENT

A 75-year-old man reported memory problems, which he said impaired his ability to function independently. He reported that he would frequently misplace household objects and would occasionally fail to remember names of familiar people and of relatives. He mentioned that he found it difficult to go shopping and was dependent on his son to take him shopping for groceries. He lived independently, looked after his personal needs. However, he needed help with chores around the house. He did admit that while he was able to buy groceries from the local store, his son looked after his finances. He also had a reasonable social life but preferred to travel by taxi as he found driving his car difficult. He said he preferred a routine for his life and was coping reasonably well, with some help from his son, who visited him weekly. He resorted to maintaining detailed diaries and appointment schedules. However, he was worried that he may have dementia.

A detailed examination did not reveal major difficulties in cognition. However, he did have mild problems on diverse aspects of functioning including complex attention, new learning, language, social cognition, perceptual-motor, and executive function. He was diagnosed to have mild cognitive impairment. His diabetes and hypertension were under control with medication. The use of daily routines and memory aides were reiterated. He was advised periodic evaluation to review his cognitive function and physical health and to monitor progression of his illness to dementia.

BOX 6.6   PSYCHOSOCIAL MANAGEMENT

Psychosocial management of people with dementia is much more important than prescribing medication to improve cognitive function. The following suggestions, to be incorporated in the daily schedule and at home, will help improve the lives of people with dementia:

- Daily schedule
  - A simple and regular daily routine
  - Daily and regular attempts to orient person
  - Regular times for waking up, naps, and sleep
  - Ample time for meals, dressing, and bathing
- Communication
  - Be patient, supportive
  - Stress sense of purpose, encourage self-expression
  - Offer comfort and reassurance
  - Don't argue, criticize; offer suggestions
  - Focus on feelings, not facts

- – Emphasize process, not result
- – Engage in conversation
- – Limit distractions
- Activities
  - – Regular exercise (e.g. walking)
  - – Activities based on current ability and enjoyment
  - – Simple recreation (e.g. listening to familiar music, watching television)
  - – Simple intellectual activities (e.g. crosswords, simple puzzles)
  - – Minimize unfamiliar activities
  - – Simple instructions before activities
  - – Clear introduction of new people and tasks
  - – Simple tasks for involvement in home
  - – Activities and links to the past
  - – Flexible approach, support, and supervision for activities
  - – Assistance with difficult tasks
  - – Substitute activity for behavior
- Food
  - – Balanced diet
  - – Limit saturated fats, refined sugars, and salt
- Modifications at home
  - – Modifications to home for hearing, vision, and mobility deficits
  - – Handrails and supports for safety
  - – Access for wheelchairs
  - – Reduction, removal of obstacles/furniture to prevent falls
  - – Labeling of switches, files, and containers
  - – Simplifying clothes and accessories (e.g. using velcro and elastic for clothes)
  - – Memory aids (e.g. calendars, clocks, dairies for appointments, and lists)

Step 7. Discuss the role of stress especially on relatives

The burden of dementia on family members should be discussed. Psychological support, respite from care, counseling, and occasionally antidepressant medication may be required for relatives with a high burden of care.

Step 8. Elaborate coping strategies

A simple and regular daily routine is essential. The fact that changes in the environment and daily routine increase the confusion and the consequent difficulty need to be highlighted. Regular exercise (walking) is helpful. Simple recreation within the daily schedule is helpful. Unfamiliar activities (e.g. meeting new people, and new situations) should be minimized. The house may need to be modified to help elderly people cope with failing memory.

BOX 6.7 SCREENING FOR DEMENTIA

The burden of dementia is well recognized. The highlighting of the illness in medical literature and the popular press has resulted in an increased awareness of the syndrome. It has also resulted in increased anxiety among older people who tend to attribute age-related cognitive decline to disease. Physicians have increased their surveillance of the condition by screening individuals in the community and in primary care.

Nevertheless, issues related to routine screening and reliable diagnosis of dementia in the community is complex. Cognitive decline among older people exists on a spectrum between age-related cognitive decline at one end through mild cognitive impairment and to frank dementia at the other. The dividing line, based on clinical assessment and psychometric tests, between normal and abnormal will remain arbitrary, as a pathological diagnosis based on brain biopsy is not possible. Studies have documented that even minor changes in clinical criteria will result in wide variations in prevalence rates. Standard criteria, which are based on age, education, and cultural norms of populations, are hard to come by in many countries.

The prevalence of dementia in the community remains low (e.g. <10%). The use of routine screening in the community is fraught with difficulty, as even screening instruments with good sensitivity and specificity, result in high false-positive rates, as these values are prevalence dependent. Consequently, screening should be reserved for those who are symptomatic rather than as a routine procedure. Testing symptomatic people will artificially increase the prevalence in the population tested and will lead to fewer false-positive results.

A simple and structured daily routine for meals, bath, exercise, and bedtime needs to be in place. Labeling of switches and containers is useful. The use of memory aids, such as calendars, clocks, diaries for appointments, and lists for reminders, help. Simple instructions before activities and the introduction of new and unfamiliar people and situations are mandatory. Simplifying clothes and accessories, and using velcro and elastic go a long way in keeping people with failing abilities independent. Daily and regular attempts to orient people with dementia are necessary.

Step 9. Negotiate a treatment plan

Most patients and families expect cures from doctors and come back with the same or new complaints for the physician to resolve. The responsibility for psychosocial management must be with the family and caregivers. Compliance with the treatment regimen is crucial, as is patient and family participation in the psychosocial program and in improving coping strategies.

Step 10. Give a specific appointment for review

A regular review of the patient's condition is mandatory for fine-tuning medication, and for providing support and advice to relatives. These visits can be used to offer psychological assistance for families and to discuss alternative coping strategies.

WILL I BE ABLE TO CURE THE PATIENT'S DISEASE?

The treatment of dementia with a treatable cause (e.g. hypothyroidism, vitamin deficiencies, and substance dependence) will result in marked improvements. However, most causes of dementia are progressive and cure is not currently possible. This suggests the need to focus on delaying the course and improving coping strategies of patients and families.

WHEN SHOULD I REFER A PATIENT FOR SPECIALIST HELP?

Dementias can be managed in primary care settings. Referral may be required for special investigations available only in tertiary care and for the management of treatable dementias. Psychiatric evaluation and specialist counseling may be necessary for incapacitating behavioral and psychological symptoms.

CONCLUSION

It is necessary to recognize dementia and distinguish it from normal aging and mild cognitive impairment. Identifying specific causes and risk factors and managing them is mandatory. Instituting treatments to delay progression of the disease and managing behavioral and psychological symptoms is crucial. Most importantly, helping the family understand the importance of a good psychosocial rehabilitation program and implementing it are cardinal in the management of people with dementias. Helping relatives cope with the burden and improve their quality of life is also necessary.

7 Alcohol and Substance Use and Dependence

Alcohol and substance use and dependence is characterized by the excessive use of alcohol or subtances, withdrawal symptoms, increased tolerance, craving, salience of the substance-seeking behavior, narrowing of the drug use repertoire, and impairments in social and occupational functioning. Alcohol and substance dependence are associated with road traffic accidents, head injury, infections, and vitamin and nutritional deficiencies. The excessive use of alcohol and substances affects many systems in the body, particularly liver function.

The management of alcohol and substance dependence includes detoxification and de-addiction. Detoxification includes the identification and treatment of medical and neurological complications, management of vitamin and nutritional deficiencies, correction of electrolyte disturbance, and treatment of infections. The discontinuation of alcohol and substances and substitution with cross-tolerant drugs (e.g. benzodiazepines) or medication to reduce the impact of withdrawal is mandatory. The de-addiction process involves the identification of cues for substance use and the discussion of changes in philosophy, attitude, and lifestyle.

INTRODUCTION

Humans have been using a variety of substances and methods to alter states of mind. While some approaches have social sanction (e.g. coffee and tea), other approaches are deemed illegal (e.g. opioids). While many people use socially sanctioned mind-altering substances (e.g. coffee and alcohol) in moderation, others use the substances in quantities and patterns, which results in serious health and social consequences.

Many people who are at risk for, or who are already experiencing, alcohol or substance-related social and medical problems receive their healthcare from primary care physicians rather than psychiatrists. Consequently, primary care settings offer an important opportunity to identify and treat people with drinking and substance-related problems. Brief interventions and counseling delivered by general practitioners (GPs) can be successful for many people. In fact, those with milder forms of addiction, which have a better prognosis, are much more amenable to change through GP intervention than psychiatric interventions, which are often provided to those with chronic use, substance dependence with serious health consequences. This chapter discusses a simple approach to managing people with alcohol and substance use problems attending primary care.

How common is alcohol use in primary care?

Alcohol use is common across regions and cultures. The prevalence of alcohol use disorders varies across nations, cultures, ethnicity, regions, age, and gender. It also varies based on governmental policies related to taxation, licensing, and advertising.

What is the recommended limit for alcohol use?

The recommended maximum intake of alcohol is 14 units a week for men and for women. (The previous recommendation was 21 units a week for men.) There is also an increased risk of harmful effects of alcohol if more than 5–7 units are consumed on a single occasion. No level of alcohol is safe during pregnancy.

A rough guide to calculating units of alcohol is:
1 unit = 10 ml or 8 grams of pure alcohol = small glass [125 ml] of 9% wine = 25 mL of 40% spirits = half pint of 3.5% beer.

What are the common patterns of alcohol use seen in primary care?

Patterns of alcohol use seen in primary care include:

- drinking that is not associated with risks (i.e. less than 14 units per week spread over 3–4 days).
- use that has resulted in physical disease or psychiatric problems
- a state in which alcohol has become central to the person's life, with a loss of control over the habit and an inability to cut down on its use.

What are the common challenges in treating problem drinking in primary care?

The physician faces a number of challenges with regard to injudicious use of alcohol:

- identifying the excessive drinker
- convincing the patient that there is a problem, which must be addressed
- detoxification in the dependent patient
- encouraging control, abstinence, or prevention of relapse.

What happens to patients who do not get help from physicians?

The complications of alcohol use are many and include:

- *Medical Problems* – hepatitis, cirrhosis, gastritis, portal hypertension, pancreatitis, ascites, aspiration pneumonia
- *Neurological Problems* – poor memory, seizures, delirium, dementia, neuropathy
- *Psychiatric Syndromes* – psychosis, depression, anxiety
- *Accidents or Injuries* due to alcohol use
- *Legal and Social Problems* – marital problems, domestic violence, child abuse or neglect, absenteeism, and problems at work.

WHAT ARE THE DIFFERENCES BETWEEN PATIENTS ATTENDING A PSYCHIATRIC HOSPITAL AND THOSE WHO PRESENT TO PRIMARY CARE?

Patients with alcohol problems seen in primary care are often those with early and mild problems. They use alcohol above the recommended limit of 14 units per week or excessive use of over 5–7 units per occasion and do not have major physical or psychiatric complications. On the other hand, people attending psychiatric facilities have patterns of use suggesting dependence with major physical and psychiatric complications. People with milder alcohol use patterns are usually more receptive to education than those with established dependence patterns of drinking who present to psychiatrists. Their motivation to stop or cut down the habit may be better than those who present late to specialists.

HOW DO PATIENTS WHO ATTEND PRIMARY CARE MANIFEST THEIR ALCOHOL-RELATED PROBLEMS?

Alcohol use comes in many forms. It is frequently hidden and often denied. Injudicious use of alcohol predisposes a person to accidents, and marital, social, and legal problems. People with problem drinking often present for other medical problems but may report sleep disturbance, tremor, and irritability. Occasionally, they may also report marital discord, anxiety, or depression. Patients in primary care may also present in states of intoxication or in a withdrawal state following total or relative abstinence from alcohol. They may, on questioning, admit to alcohol use, especially to induce sleep. The patient and/or his family may also present with distress secondary to the social or legal problems that have occurred as a result of alcohol use.

Excessive consumption of alcohol may go unnoticed until the alcohol is removed, perhaps in hospital. Admission for surgery or to a coronary care unit may precipitate withdrawal. The withdrawal syndrome may not be recognized and it is imperative to be aware of the possibility as a differential diagnosis.

IS THERE A QUICK WAY TO SCREEN FOR PROBLEM DRINKING?

There are a number of questionnaires that can be used to assess alcohol use and dependence. A simple instrument, known by its mnemonic CAGE, is often used to screen for problem drinking.

- Have you ever thought of **C**utting down on your drinking?
- Have you ever been **A**nnoyed by people telling you to cut down on your drinking?
- Have you ever felt **G**uilty about your drinking?
- Do you need a drink in the morning to get you going (an **E**ye-opener)?

If two or more of the CAGE questions are answered in the affirmative, then the specificity is around 90%. It is likely that the patient has an alcohol problem and there are very few false-positive results. The sensitivity is much lower and many with an alcohol use disorder will be missed. Three positive responses raise the specificity to nearly 100%, but at the expense of reducing the sensitivity to less than 50%.

Unexpected laboratory results, such as macrocytosis on complete blood counts or elevated enzymes on liver function tests, should also alert clinicians to the possibility of problem drinking.

How should I elicit the details?

It is essential to take a history in a non-confrontational and non-judgmental manner, documenting past alcohol use, binge drinking, and the effects of alcohol on the person's behavior. Does the patient use alcohol in risky situations, such as driving a vehicle or operating machinery? Does drinking result in failure to meet family and social obligations? Have there been unsuccessful attempts to cut down? Have there been symptoms of withdrawal in the past?

What are the common presenting problems of excessive use?

People with problem drinking often ingest alcohol in larger amounts or over a longer period than they intended. Craving, the strong and persistent desire to drink, and unsuccessful attempts at cutting down or controlling alcohol consumption is common. Increased time spent in attempting to obtain the substance, using it, and recovering from its effects are characteristic. The failure to meet obligations at school/work and at home and continued use even in the presence of physical, psychological, social, and occupational impairment is indicative of problem drinking. Recurrent use in situations in which it is physically hazardous is not uncommon. The development of tolerance to the effects of alcohol and withdrawal symptoms, when abstinent, are also symptomatic of problem drinking.

How do I make a diagnosis?

The diagnosis essentially involves the recognition of the pattern of alcohol use. The traditional patterns that suggest problem drinking includes harmful use (harmful use is defined as drinking that results in physical or mental damage).

Dependence states are characterized by the following:

- a strong desire to consume alcohol
- difficulty in controling its use
- withdrawal features such as insomnia, anxiety, tremors, and sweating when alcohol use is ceased
- tolerance or drinking large amounts of alcohol without appearing intoxicated
- continued use despite harmful consequences
- neglect of other activities due to alcohol; social and occupational impairment.

More recent diagnostic criteria argue for diagnostic categories called substance use disorder, when more than one of the symptoms listed is present.

Intoxication is a transient state following the use of alcohol that results in a disturbance in the level of consciousness, thinking, mood, perception, and behavior (which may vary from agitation and aggression to social withdrawal and sedation). It is commonly associated with slurred speech, incoordination, unsteady gait, nystagmus, and impairment in attention and memory. Occasionally, it can present as stupor or coma. The intensity lessens with time and eventually disappears in the absence of further use.

Withdrawal develops following an absolute or relative reduction in the consumption of alcohol after repeated and prolonged use. The symptoms of withdrawal may include autonomic hyperactivity (sweating, rapid heart rate >100 beats per minute), increased hand tremor, insomnia, nausea, vomiting, elevated temperature, increased blood pressure, restlessness, agitation, anxiety, psychosis, seizures, and rarely even death.

Delirium following the withdrawal of alcohol is also called delirium tremens. This is a medical emergency as it can be life-threatening. It usually occurs within the first 48–72 hours of alcohol withdrawal. The symptoms that occur include clouding of consciousness and confusion, vivid hallucinations and illusions (most commonly visual and auditory), and tremors. The other symptoms that may occur include insomnia, agitation, fearfulness, and suspicion.

WHAT ARE THE STEPS OF THE SUGGESTED MANAGEMENT PROTOCOL?

The ten steps in management are:

1. Recognize the clinical presentation
2. Acknowledge distress
3. Elicit the patient's and the family's perspective
4. Take a focused history; carry out physical examination and laboratory investigations to rule out medical problems
5. Educate the patient about the nature of illness and its treatment
6. Prescribe medication
7. Discuss the role of stress as cause and consequence of illness
8. Elaborate coping strategies
9. Negotiate a treatment plan, compliance, participation, and responsibility
10. Give an appointment for review.

Step 1. Recognize the clinical presentation

Substance use and dependence should be considered in situations where the patient presents with sleep disturbance, occupational problems, marital discord, road traffic accidents, and medical complications of alcohol (i.e. liver dysfunction). The first step is an assessment of the habit. The duration of the habit, the amount regularly consumed, and the pattern of drinking need to be examined to determine the nature of problem drinking.

Step 2. Acknowledge distress

The distress of the person and particularly of the family members should be acknowledged. This helps in establishing rapport, conveying empathy, and starting a therapeutic relationship.

Step 3. Elicit the patient's and the family's perspective

Eliciting patient and family perspectives about the habit will provide insights into the situation. It can also serve to identify stress, which may be contributing to the alcohol use: marital discord, interpersonal problems, sexual difficulties, work-related difficulties, financial burden, debt, etc. The admission that sleep disturbance is the cause of the habit will suggest that withdrawal symptoms are making it a vicious cycle and that there is a need to break it using benzodiazepine medication. Eliciting the patient's perspective will also provide insights into the motivation of the patient to quit the habit. The extent of family problems and support can also be gauged.

Step 4. Take a focused history; carry out physical examination and laboratory investigations

A focused history and physical examination, including neurological examination, is cardinal to identify alcohol-related problems, including liver disease, vitamin deficiencies, injuries, and peripheral neuropathies. A mental state assessment of the level of consciousness, orientation to time, place and person, attention, concentration, and the presence or absence of psychotic, anxiety or depressive symptoms is mandatory. Medical investigations should be ordered to assess general health, diabetic status, and kidney and liver functions (Table 7.1).

Step 5. Educate the patient about the illness and treatment

Educate the patient about the various harmful effects of alcohol, including physical, psychological, and social issues. Provide feedback by linking, when appropriate, the alcohol use to existing medical problems (such as hypertension or gastritis), abnormal blood tests (LFT or elevated blood sugars), or psychosocial problems (marital or work-related). Discuss the biochemical basis of developing tolerance and withdrawal symptoms, and discuss habit formation over time.

Step 6. Medical management

Patients need to be assessed for vitamin deficiencies, dehydration, injuries, and infections. Frank thiamine deficiency is rare but many people dependent on alcohol will have low reserves of the vitamin, which places them at risk for complications such as delirium tremens, encephalopathy, and psychosis. Vitamin supplements for those whose dietary intake of vitamins has been poor is mandatory. As oral thiamine is poorly absorbed, parenteral thiamine should be given if low reserves are suspected. Tetanus toxoid should be given to those with injuries. Infections and electrolyte disturbances should be managed.

The immediate management of alcohol withdrawal is called detoxification. Patients with moderate withdrawal symptoms may require benzodiazepines (Table 7.2). Most can be detoxified as outpatients or at home. Chlordiazepoxide or lorazepam is recommended. People who drink only in the evenings can receive small bedtime doses

---

TABLE 7.1

Investigations to be Considered in the Assessment of Patients Presenting with Alcohol Use

- Electrolytes (especially in patients who are disoriented and in delirium)
- Full blood examination
- Liver function tests
- Serum creatinine, blood sugars (if patient above 40 years of age).

TABLE 7.2

Some Common Medications Used in the Treatment of Alcohol Use

Medication	Starting dose	Adult dose	Common side-effects	Indications	Duration of treatment
Chlordiazepoxide (long-acting benzodiazepine)	10–20 mg	40–120 mg (divided doses)	Sedation, falls in the elderly	Alcohol withdrawal	Administer the drug every 4–6 hours. Adjust the dose and frequency based on severity of the withdrawal symptoms. Taper gradually, every day or alternate day, by 10 mg / 1 mg on the basis of reduction in symptoms
Lorazepam (short-acting benzodiazepine)	1–2 mg	8–10 mg (divided doses)	Sedation, falls in the elderly	Alcohol withdrawal, specifically for those with significant liver disease that might impair their ability to metabolize a long-acting agent	
Haloperidol (first generation antipsychotic)	1.0–2.5 mg	5–10 mg	Extra-pyramidal symptoms, dystonia, akathisia, tardive dyskinesia	Agitation, psychosis, delirium tremens; given as intramuscular injection for severely disturbed patients	If given for withdrawal-related psychotic symptoms, gradually taper after 4–5 months without symptoms.
Risperidone (newer antipsychotic)	1 mg	2–4 mg	Extra-pyramidal symptoms (less than with haloperidol), dystonia, akathisia, tardive dyskinesia	Agitation, psychotic symptoms, delirium tremens	In case of persisting psychosis after detoxification, long-term use may be indicated

of 10–30 mg of chlordiazepoxide (5–15 mg of diazepam or 1–3 mg of lorazepam). Higher and divided doses will be necessary for those who have been drinking in the morning or those with withdrawal symptoms that occur in the daytime. Doses of 40–80 mg per day of chlordiazepoxide, divided and given three or four times a day, may be needed.

Dispensing should be daily and must be supervised by family members to prevent the risk of misuse or overdose. Daily supervision is essential in the first few days; frequent follow-ups are advisable thereafter to adjust the dose of medication, assess whether the patient has returned to drinking, check for serious withdrawal symptoms and maintain support. The dose can be gradually tapered and stopped over 7–15 days after the withdrawal symptoms have subsided.

Step 7. Identification of cues for drinking and stressors

Helping the patient to identify high-risk situations in which drinking is likely to occur or cues for drinking, such as family celebrations, spending time in the company of friends who consume alcohol or stressful situations at work, is necessary. Discuss with the patient techniques and healthy alternatives for managing such high-risk situations. Regular and frequent meals, the control of money, staying away from bars and liquor shops and developing healthy leisure activities are useful techniques. The presence of a supportive network of friends, family and the doctor will help in this process.

The identification of stress, which has precipitated, exacerbated or maintained the habit is necessary. Marital discord, interpersonal problems, sexual difficulties, work-related difficulties, financial burden, debt, etc. can be cited as examples to see if the patient and family admit to similar problems.

Step 8. Counseling for specific problems

General solutions for improving mental health, including yoga, meditation, physical exercise, leisure and religion (if the person is religious), are useful measures. Patients with specific problems, such as marital discord, work-related issues, or financial problems, would need help with problem solving. Asking patients to look for specific solutions for their difficulties and giving them time to examine the issues are obligatory.

The realization that it is not the physician's responsibility to solve the patient's alcohol dependence and that he can only empower patients to resolve it themselves comes with experience. The specific solutions to the problem have to be the patient's own. The physician's role is to empower the patient and the family.

Step 9. Negotiate a treatment plan, compliance, participation and responsibility

Excessive alcohol use is a habit, which causes physical disease and psychological and social problems. The physician's responsibility is to manage withdrawal symptoms and detoxification, and discuss strategies for preventing relapse of the habit. Emphasizing that change in the habit is the patient's responsibility and that only he/she him/herself can make a decision to change and make life better is mandatory. Since alcohol use is often associated with a certain lifestyle, giving up the habit requires a change in philosophy, attitude and that particular way of life.

Step 10. Follow-up and reinforcement

To ensure the long-term effectiveness of the brief intervention described above, ensure regular follow-up visits with the patient and reinforce the abstinent behavior. Anxiety and depression often co-occur with alcohol misuse. The patient may have been using alcohol to self-medicate to reduce these symptoms. If symptoms such as sleep disturbance, stress, and depression persist for more than 2 weeks following detoxification, treatment with antidepressants and counseling should be considered.

BOX 7.1 A NOTE ON THE MANAGEMENT OF DELIRIUM TREMENS

Delirium tremens is a medical emergency. Hospitalization is recommended. In patients who are in withdrawal, dehydration should be corrected and infections treated as these can precipitate the condition. Frequent monitoring of the pulse rate, blood pressure, respiration, and level of consciousness are important. Ensure adequate hydration and nutrition. Intramuscular thiamine must be administered once a day for a few days if you suspect the possibility of deficiency; oral supplements of vitamin B complex and thiamine (100 mg daily) must also be given. Higher parenteral doses are required if the patient has features of Wernicke encephalopathy/Korsakoff psychosis. Treat injuries with tetanus toxoid and antibiotics, if required. Keep the patient in an evenly lit, quiet room, where dark shadows, bright lights, loud noises, and other excessive stimuli are avoided.

Patients with severe dependence and a history of withdrawal seizures and delirium tremens require doses of up to 100–120 mg equivalent of chlordiazepoxide (i.e. 50–60 mg of diazepam or 10–12 mg of lorazepam). This requires close supervision and adjustment, based on the severity of the patient's withdrawal symptoms and response to medication. For patients in withdrawal delirium, antipsychotic drugs in low doses can be used along with the benzodiazepines to reduce agitation. Anticonvulsant medication can also be added in patients with a history of recurrent withdrawal seizures.

BOX 7.2 A NOTE ON MANAGING OTHER SUBSTANCE USE AND DEPENDENCE

People who abuse other substances and are dependent on them can also be managed with this protocol. Small doses of chlorpromazine and benzodiazepines can be used for detoxification. Antipsychotics can also be used to control severe restlessness and agitation. Severe withdrawal and dependence may require hospitalization and treatment. Opioid withdrawal may require substitution with appropriate agents. Mild withdrawal can be managed with antipsychotic medication.

The following situations may require specialist help:

- Hospital detoxification is recommended in patients at risk for complicated withdrawal syndrome (with a current or past history of seizures or delirium tremens).
- Patients with multiple drug use or dependence and those with a severe comorbid medical or psychiatric disorder.
- Patients who are at a significant risk of suicide may also require specialist input and likely inpatient detoxification.
- Ataxia, confusion, memory disturbance, delirium tremens, hypothermia and hypotension, ophthalmoplegia, or unconsciousness mandate hospitalization and specialist help.
- Non-urgent referral to a mental health specialist may be required if there is a severe

---

BOX 7.3 A NOTE ON THE PROGNOSIS

Once alcohol or substance use becomes a habit and leads to dependence, the prognosis for complete abstinence is relatively poor. However, many patients are able to cut down the amount of alcohol. There is no magic formula for treatment; some intervention is better than no intervention and different types of interventions seem to have similar outcomes. Consequently, GPs can play a major role in reducing alcohol and substance intake and in preventing relapse. Those who relapse should be encouraged to be admitted for a detoxification and de-addiction package. Even if complete abstinence is not possible, reduction of the amount and the time spent under the influence of alcohol helps many people.

BOX 7.4 ALCOHOL DEPENDENCE

A 40-year-old man presented with a two-day history of severe abdominal discomfort. On enquiry he mentioned a 10-year history of alcohol use. He also mentioned that for the past five years, he had to consume alcohol daily as he had sleep disturbance and tremors of his hands if he did not drink. He had increased the quantity of alcohol consumption over the past few years. His habit was a cause of marital discord. He was also frequently unable to go for work.

He was diagnosed to have alcoholic gastritis and alcohol dependence. He was started on tab. omeprazole, 20 mg twice a day, for his gastritis. He was educated about the nature of his problem. He was prescribed tab. chlordiazepoxide, 10 mg in the morning and 40 mg at bedtime. This medication was tapered over the next 10 days. He was also given parenteral and oral vitamins and thiamine. Cues which led to his drinking were identified and he was advised alternative strategies to manage them.

mental illness, or if symptoms of mental illness persist after detoxification and abstinence.
- Referral may be considered to commence agents such as naltrexone and disulfiram, which may be useful in prolonging abstinence.

BOX 7.5   DELIRIUM TREMENS

A 50-year-old man presented with a four-day history of fear, persecutory ideas, sleep disturbance, restlessness, and agitation. On enquiry, he mentioned that he had reduced his intake of alcohol a week ago. He reported a 20-year history of alcohol use. For the past 10 years, he had been consuming alcohol every day and had also started drinking in the morning for the past year. The quantity of alcohol consumed had increased over the past few years. His habit was also a cause of marital discord and he had lost his job. On examination, the patient was disoriented to time, place, and person. He mentioned persecutory delusions and was observed to have marked tremors of his hands. His liver function tests revealed moderate elevation of enzymes.

He was diagnosed to have delirium tremens and alcohol dependence. The patient was prescribed tab. chlordiazepoxide, 100 mg in three divided doses. This medication was tapered over 10 days. He was also given parenteral and oral vitamins and thiamine. He was educated about the nature of his problems. Cues that led to his drinking were identified and he was advised alternative strategies to deal with them. Detailed discussions were held on the need for him to give up his habit and change his philosophy, lifestyle, and attitude.

BOX 7.6   CANNABIS USE COMPLICATING CHRONIC PSYCHOSIS

A 20-year-old college student was brought by his parents to a primary care clinic. They reported deteriorating academic performance and social withdrawal. They also mentioned that he was abusing cannabis for the past year. An assessment suggested that the student was "hearing voices" and was convinced that his friends and family members would harm him. He started experimenting with cannabis and reported a temporary reduction in his distress. However, he mentioned apathy and social withdrawal resulted in absence from college and deteriorating academic performance.

A detailed evaluation suggested a diagnosis of chronic psychosis. He was started on risperidone and the dose gradually increased to 6 mg per day. His symptoms of psychosis, abnormal beliefs, and auditory hallucinations gradually subsided. He was educated about the risks of using cannabis as it could worsen the psychosis in the long term. He was advised to let go of his drug habit after his psychotic symptoms responded to psychotropic medication.

OTHER SUBSTANCE USE DISORDERS

Humans abuse a variety of substances. While the use of alcohol is common, many other substances are routinely employed for recreational use and to relieve distress. The development of withdrawal symptoms and tolerance leads to addiction and chronic use.

The substances commonly used include: tobacco (e.g. cigarettes, chewing tobacco, and snuff), caffeine (e.g. from coffee, tea, caffeinated drinks, and energy drinks), cannabis, hallucinogens (e.g. phencyclidine), inhalant use (e.g. glues, paints, fuels, and other volatile compounds), opioids (e.g. morphine and heroin), and stimulants (e.g. amphetamine and cocaine). Sedatives, hypnotics, anxiolytics, and pain medications can also be commonly misused, with the development of dependence.

The clinical characteristics and diagnostic criteria for substance use disorders due to different substances are similar to those used to establish alcohol use and dependence. They report ingestion of larger amounts of substances or over a longer period than they intended. Craving, the strong and persistent desire to use the substance, and the unsuccessful attempts at cutting down or controling consumption is common. Increased time spent in attempting to obtain the substance, using it, and recovering from its effects are characteristic. The failure to meet obligations at school/work and at home and continued use even in the presence of physical, psychological, social, and occupational impairment is indicative of substance abuse. Recurrent use in situations in which it is physically hazardous is not uncommon. The development of tolerance to the effects of the substance and withdrawal symptoms, when abstinent, are also symptomatic of substance use and dependence.

Caffeine withdrawal is characterized by headache, fatigue, dysphoria, drowsiness,

---

BOX 7.7   CHRONIC BENZODIAZEPINE USE

A 50-year-old homemaker, who had recently moved into the neighborhood, presented to her GP. She requested a prescription for alprazolam as she has been using it for many years. She said that she was an anxious and sensitive person, who was easily upset by day-to-day events. However, she mentioned that she had coped for the past few years by using medication prescribed by her previous family doctor. The drug calmed her down quickly and she began to slowly increase the dose, as it effects wore off rapidly. She felt that she did not have any stress in her life but admitted to having difficulty falling asleep.

The GP discussed her anxious personality traits and her dependence on medication to cope with life. He educated her about withdrawal symptoms and increasing tolerance. He substituted the alprazolam with longer-acting benzodiazepine clonazepam and then gradually tapered it over time. He also prescribed a small dose of a sedative antidepressant. He encouraged the patient to consider alternative stress reduction and coping strategies such as yoga, meditation, and physical exercise. She was able to come off the benzodiazepines within four weeks and the antidepressants over the next 12 months.

BOX 7.8   PUBLIC HEALTH POLICIES AND ALCOHOL USE

There is increasing recognition that consumption of alcohol is a major contributor to the burden of disease in many nations, particularly those categorized as low- and middle-income countries. Morbidity and mortality due to alcohol is a major public health concern. Extreme policies of prohibition are counterproductive as they are impossible to enforce and result in bootlegging, sale of illicit and unregulated alcohol, associated crime, and loss of tax revenue. On the other hand, governments addicted to the taxes from the sale of alcohol allow permissive strategies to increase revenue.

The complex relationships between policies, economics, and politics of alcohol and public health and between governments, industry, and individuals call for a thorough review of the complex situation. While public health implications of policies concerning alcohol have long been accepted, the failure to implement many of these policies demands a more balanced and nuanced approach to the problem that integrates both the regulation of availability of alcohol as well as helps in rigorously enforcing the law.

and difficulty in concentration, while tobacco withdrawal should be suspected when people report irritability, anger, frustration, depression, increased appetite, and insomnia. Withdrawal from cannabis often results in irritability, anxiety, sleep disturbance, reduced appetite, depressed mood, and restlessness. People with stimulant withdrawal present with fatigue, unpleasant dreams, agitation or psychomotor retardation, and increased or reduced sleep. Those with opioid withdrawal report nausea, vomiting, diarrhea, muscle aches, lacrimation, sweating, insomnia, yawning, fever, piloerection, dysphoria, and pupillary dilatation.

Intoxication with substance should always be suspected when people come to emergency departments of hospitals. They often present with autonomic dysfunction (e.g. tachycardia, hypertension, sweating, and palpitations), neurological signs (e.g. nystagmus, ataxia, dysarthria, diminished response to pain, numbness, blurred vision, and hyperacusis), seizures, and coma. Stimulant and hallucinogen intoxication presents with pupillary dilatation, while opioid intoxication presents with pupillary constriction.

The principles of detoxification are similar to that employed for alcohol. A high index of suspicion will facilitate the identification of the clinical presentation. Stimulant and hallucinogen intoxication are medical emergencies and should be managed in hospital. Identification and management of infections, injuries, electrolyte disturbance, blood pressure, seizures, and nutritional deficiencies are crucial.

Substitution with appropriate cross-tolerant medication is necessary. However, benzodiazepine and antipsychotic medication can also be used in opioid and stimulant withdrawal.

De-addiction therapy is also similar to that employed for alcohol problems. Unconditional positive regard for the person and a non-judgmental relationship is cardinal to establishing a therapeutic relationship. The identification of cues, their substitution with other more constructive activities, and the management of stress are necessary. The need to change personality, attitude, and lifestyle will require that the person accept responsibility for his/her behavior and life. Long-term support is crucial for abstinence.

Recurrent relapses, severe, and intractable use may require hospitalization and specialist referral. Similarly, persistent psychiatric and neurological complications, and significant marital discord, will need referral.

CONCLUSION

A GP can conduct brief interventions for the treatment of alcohol and substance use with a focused physical examination, ensuring adequate general medical care, using benzodiazepines or other medication for detoxification, providing education about ill-effects of alcohol and substances used, helping the patient to accept responsibility, identify triggers for his behavior, and attempt problem-solving for life stressors. In many cases, if the GP has had a long-term and trusting relationship with the patient, she or he can play an important role in influencing the patient to change his/her behavior.

8 Psychosis

Psychoses are characterized by the presence of strange beliefs (delusions), hearing voices, or seeing visions in the absence of stimuli (hallucinations), and grossly abnormal behavior. They are also associated with disturbed sleep, loss of appetite, poor personal care, preoccupation, social withdrawal or restlessness, and agitation. Problems in attention and concentration, lack of motivation, apathy, and poor work performance can also be present. Psychoses can be classified as acute and chronic, and as episodic or continuous.

The management of psychotic disturbance involves the use of antipsychotic medication. The medication has to be continued for about two years to prevent relapses in those with an episode of acute psychosis. People with chronic psychosis will require treatment and prophylaxis for a much longer period. Psychosocial management is essential to recovery and rehabilitation.

INTRODUCTION

Psychotic syndromes are seen infrequently in general practice and general hospital settings. Nevertheless, when they do occasionally present, it is important to be able to identify and manage them appropriately. This chapter describes the management of people who present with psychosis to general practice settings.

WHAT ARE THE KINDS OF PRESENTATIONS OF PSYCHOSES IN GENERAL HOSPITAL SETTINGS?

The two common presentations of psychosis in general medical settings are:

- Disturbed and violent patients, those with acute presentation or episodic illness
- Patients with a history of psychosis who present with apathy, social withdrawal, and are unable to hold a job.

WHAT USUALLY HAPPENS TO SUCH PATIENTS IN GENERAL HOSPITAL SETTINGS?

The patients who are disturbed or violent (i.e. with acute psychosis and psychotic exacerbations) are often given benzodiazepines and referred to psychiatric services. Those with chronic psychosis, apathy, social withdrawal, and residual symptoms are often missed.

Social stigma is often associated with mental illness. It often results in discrimination in society and in the workplace. Despite a revolution in psychiatry, significant advance in psychotropic medication, many changes in psychiatric practice, and the increasing number of people who benefit from treatment, psychiatric diagnosis continues to be stigmatizing. Consequently, many people are hesitant to seek psychiatric help and intervention. Their refusal to go to psychiatric facilities results in their not receiving treatment for their distressing conditions. Even those patients who are forced to go to psychiatric centers during acute episodes and exacerbations of psychosis refuse to continue with treatment due to the stigma of mental illness. Consequently, many people with psychosis who would benefit from psychiatric treatment and services have a low level of compliance with psychotropic medication and therapy, and continue to have distressing symptoms and a poorer quality of life than they would otherwise have had, had they been on psychiatric treatment. The shortage of specialists and the high costs of tertiary care also add to their difficulties.

WHAT ARE THE COMMON SYMPTOMS OF PSYCHOSIS?

The key features that define psychotic disorders are delusions, hallucinations, disorganized or grossly abnormal speech, behavior, and negative symptoms. Delusions are fixed beliefs that are not amenable to change in the light of contradictory evidence. Such beliefs include: persecutory (of harm, or harassment), referential (certain gestures, comments, and environmental cues are directed at oneself), grandiose (belief in their exceptional abilities, wealth, or fame), nihilistic (conviction of impending catastrophe), erotomanic (false belief that another person is in love with him/her), and somatic (focus on health and organ function). Delusions are deemed bizarre if they are implausible, not understandable by the person's cultural peers, or are not derived from ordinary life experiences. Beliefs about loss of control over the mind and body are generally considered bizarre (e.g. thought withdrawal, thought insertion, delusions of control). A delusion is distinguished from a strongly held belief based on the conviction, the evidence, the explanation, and the person's actions based on such opinions.

Hallucinations are perceptions that occur without an external stimulus. They are often perceived through the sense organ (e.g. ear, eye, or tongue), vivid and clear, occur in clear consciousness and are not under voluntary control. However, hallucinations occurring while falling asleep or waking up, after physical exhaustion or sleep deprivation, as part of a religious experience, and in certain cultural contexts are within the normal range of human experience.

Speech, reflecting the person's thinking, is considered abnormal, if the person moves from one topic to another, is incoherent or tangential. Grossly abnormal or disorganized behavior includes unpredictable agitation or markedly diminished reactivity to the environment and stupor. The term "negative symptoms" is used to describe diminished emotions, reduced self-motivation, decreased speech, and markedly lessened social interactions, and an inability to experience pleasure from previously pleasurable stimuli.

Psychotic disorders include those with single and circumscribed delusional beliefs (delusional disorder) and abnormal beliefs associated with hallucinations, motor disturbances, disorders of speech and behavior, and negative symptoms (schizophrenia). They can be acute (brief psychosis), episodic (schizophrenia or as part of bipolar disorders), or chronic (schizophrenia).

WHAT IS THE PREVALENCE OF PSYCHOSES?

The lifetime risk of severe mental illness (schizophrenia and bipolar disorder) is considered 1%–2%. However, there may be regional variations and differential risk within families.

WHAT IS THE ROLE OF GENERAL PHYSICIANS WORKING IN GENERAL HOSPITAL SETTINGS IN THE TREATMENT OF PSYCHOSIS?

General practitioners (GPs) can play an important role in the management of psychosis. This includes:

- the early detection of the symptoms of psychosis
- the provision of care in the low-stigma environment of general medical settings
- the provision of psychological and technical support for relatives of patients with psychotic illness.

These factors will not only help in early recognition and early institution of treatment, but can also help in improving compliance with treatment in those with chronic illness.

The specialist perspective related to diagnosis and the sub-classification of psychotic syndromes are more difficult to employ when applied in primary care and general medical settings. For example, when people with acute psychotic presentations are brought to general medical settings, these clinical conditions of short duration are difficult to sub-classify into schizophrenia or bipolar disorder. It is difficult to give the condition a specific label.

Patients with disturbed behavior and violence are difficult to interview, making it difficult to document the classical symptoms listed in the traditional psychiatric categories. The diagnosis of people who present with residual psychotic symptoms is also difficult to make based on current clinical examination as the classical signs and symptoms have often occurred in the past.

The acute psychotic presentations of schizophrenia and mania have many symptoms in common: sleep disturbance, restlessness, agitation, tendency to wander, anger, irritability, delusions, and hallucinations. This makes differentiation difficult. However, over time and with repeated assessments and consultations, the classic patterns may become obvious. Nevertheless, the general protocol will help manage these patients without specifically diagnosing a particular psychiatric disorder. The protocol is simple and is flexible, so that it allows specific and additional treatments, which may be appropriate. This module helps one to recognize the pattern of illness and manage it. It does not focus on labels or sub-classification, such as schizophrenia, mania, or delusional disorder.

IF A SINGLE PROTOCOL IS USEFUL, WHY ARE THERE SO MANY DIFFERENT MANAGEMENT GUIDELINES?

Many of these guidelines are derived from specialist settings and may be useful for patients with severe and chronic disease. They may not be necessary for patients who present to primary care and to general medical and surgical practice facilities. In addition, different protocols are complex and often not easily employable in the primary care settings by physicians and GPs.

The suggested protocol has been developed in collaboration with general physicians over a period of many years. The protocol has been modified over time to incorporate important psychiatric and physician principles. The steps, the sequence and their rationale are briefly described.

WHAT ARE THE TEN STEPS?

The ten steps in management are:

1. Recognize the clinical presentation
2. Acknowledge distress
3. Elicit the patient's and the family's perspective
4. Take a focused history; carry out physical examination and laboratory investigations to rule out medical problems
5. Educate the patient about the nature of illness and its treatment
6. Prescribe medication
7. Discuss the role of stress as cause and consequence of illness
8. Elaborate coping strategies
9. Negotiate a treatment plan, compliance, participation, and responsibility
10. Give an appointment for review.

Step 1. Recognize clinical presentation – identify the psychotic syndrome

A psychotic illness is characterized by a loss of contact with reality, as evidenced by the presence of strange beliefs (delusions), hearing voices/seeing visions (hallucinations), incoherent speech, and grossly abnormal behavior (Box 8.1).

These problems cause significant difficulty in coping with the demands of daily life. The syndrome can be established by taking a careful history and confirmed by clinical examination. Relatives will often give a history of behavioral changes, such as restlessness, irritability, suspicions, fear, talking or smiling even in the absence of other people, bizarre behavior, and disjointed speech (positive symptoms).

Some patients may present with neglect of personal care, reduced speech, decreased interest and performance in occupational and academic activities, and social withdrawal (negative symptoms). Others may report slowness in thinking, inability to plan, and reduced concentration and memory (cognitive symptoms).

Useful questions to elicit symptoms during examination include, "Have you recently had the feeling that people are talking about you or plotting to harm you?", "Is there anything special about you that may make anyone want to do that?", "Have there been times when you have heard voices or seen things when no one else was around and there was nothing else to explain it?".

Psychotic symptoms of less than four-weeks' duration are termed as acute psychotic episode. Chronic psychosis, on the other hand, is characterized by a longer duration of psychotic symptoms and may be sub-classified into schizophrenia (associated with deterioration in functioning), affective psychosis (associated with mania or depression), and delusional disorders (single delusions with good functioning).

BOX 8.1   SOME CLINICAL DESCRIPTIONS

Delusions: A delusion is a false belief that the patient continues to hold despite evidence to the contrary and in spite of it not being shared by others in the same community. Delusions may be persecutory, grandiose, or bizarre in nature; sometimes they may have themes of guilt or loss.

Hallucinations: A hallucination is the experience of a perception in the absence of a sensory stimulus. It can occur in any sensory modality; auditory hallucinations are a common and often frequent symptom of psychosis.

Positive Symptoms: Delusions, hallucinations, grossly abnormal behavior, and disordered thinking and speech are often referred to as the positive symptoms of schizophrenia since they appear to reflect an excess or distortion of normal functions.

Negative Symptoms: Negative symptoms relate to those abilities or personality traits that are "lost" with schizophrenia. They may remain even during periods of remission of the positive psychotic symptoms. These symptoms include social withdrawal, not talking or making only short statements, extreme apathy, lack of drive or initiative, needing encouragement to do most tasks that other people do on their own, such as eating, bathing, or grooming, and emotional unresponsiveness.

Extrapyramidal Symptoms: Characterized by muscle rigidity, tremor, and slowness of movements, people with symptoms of drug-induced parkinsonism, or extrapyramidal symptoms may appear to have fixed facial expressions and slurred speech. These occur more commonly with the use of the older antipsychotics, such as chlorpromazine and haloperidol. The symptoms appear within days of starting medication, but usually improve within 3 months of treatment. The symptoms reduce with tab. trihexyphenidyl, 2–6 mg per day.

Dystonia: Dystonia is the sustained contraction of a group of muscles most commonly involving the tongue, jaw, neck, and trunk. Spasms are sometimes painful and can be frightening. Acute dystonia usually occurs within one or two days of beginning treatment and is usually transient. It responds dramatically to the intramuscular injection promethazine, 25–50 mg.

Tardive Dyskinesia: This usually occurs following prolonged exposure to antipsychotic medication and presents with abnormal facial movements, such as smacking of lips, chewing, sucking, twisting of the tongue, side-to-side movements of the jaw or jerky, often purposeless limb movements. It requires reduction in the antipsychotic dosage, if possible; the addition of long-acting benzodiazepines may help. Change to a newer antipsychotic is recommended.

Akathisia: This is characterized by severe motor restlessness, resulting in an inability to remain in one place for long. It requires reduction in the antipsychotic dosage, if possible; the addition of long-acting benzodiazepines will help.

Other common clinical presentations, which need to be excluded are:

- *Delirium* – disorientation to time, place, and person of very sudden onset and short duration (of a few days)
- *Dementia* – chronic memory loss associated with deficit in complex attention, learning difficulties, and problems with memory; language and speech disorders (aphasia); perceptual and motor dysfunction (apraxia, agnosia); and loss of executive function and problems in social cognition
- *Substance Dependence* – prolonged and persistent use of substances such as alcohol, cannabis, and opioids

Step 2. Acknowledge distress

Patients may be distressed because of frightening delusions and hallucinations; relatives are often scared and puzzled by the patient's odd behavior. Acknowledging their distress reflects an empathetic attitude, and contributes to establishing an effective rapport and forming a therapeutic alliance, which are essential in facilitating improvement.

Step 3. Elicit the patient's and the family's perspective

Asking patients what they think or fear is necessary for making a diagnosis, providing specific reassurance, as well as addressing issues of safety (e.g. "My wife is plotting to kill me", "I heard a message over the radio", "I will either kill her or myself before that"). Providing appropriate reassurance to the relatives is most effective if based on their actual beliefs and concerns. Therefore, it is important to understand what they think is wrong with the patient, and why this has happened to them.

Many beliefs held by patients with psychosis and their relatives contradict the biomedical model of the illness (e.g. "It could be due to black magic"). These beliefs need to be discussed and understood in their cultural context before presenting alternative biomedical explanations. The many non-medical beliefs held by the patient and relatives should not be dismissed out of hand. The biomedical explanation of the disease should be presented without belittling the patient's explanations.

Explanations of illness are also coping mechanisms used by people, their families, communities, and society. Most people seem to hold simultaneously multiple and even contradictory beliefs about disease and illness, healing and cure. The biomedical explanation of illness and the consequent need for compliance with medication and therapy need to be complementary to the use of local, cultural, and religious solutions.

Step 4. Take a focused history; carry out physical examination and laboratory investigations

It is essential to exclude medical causes and substance dependence, which may result in psychosis. Common medical causes that can result in psychosis include epilepsy, head injury, brain tumors and infections, thyroid disorders, and HIV/AIDS (Table 8.1). Alcohol and cannabis are the commonly abused substances that can give rise to psychotic symptoms.

A focused history and physical examination (especially neurological) are cardinal

TABLE 8.1

Common Physical Disorders that can Manifest with Psychotic Symptoms

- Infections (including meningitis, encephalitis, HIV)
- Cerebrovascular disease
- Head injury
- Epilepsy
- Space-occupying lesions of the central nervous system
- Thyroid disorders

to identify psychotic syndromes that are secondary to physical disease or substance use. A detailed examination of attention, concentration, orientation, and memory must be performed. Organic and substance-induced psychotic states can be differentiated from functional psychiatric disorders because they are often associated with an altered sensorium and impaired orientation, memory and concentration.

Medical investigations should be ordered (Table 8.2), not only to exclude relevant differential diagnoses, but also to assess the extent to which comorbidities such as poor nutrition and alcohol and drug use might be affecting the patient's general health. Additional investigations are necessary if the person is disoriented or confused or has progressive memory loss.

If medical and substance-induced causes are absent, then a diagnosis of acute or chronic psychosis can be made on the basis of the duration of symptoms. If medical causes or substance abuse is present, then the psychosis can be considered secondary to these conditions.

Step 5. Educate the patient and the family about the nature of illness and treatment

Inform the relatives that agitation and strange behavior are symptoms of a mental disorder, a disease of the brain; that the disease is not due to what anybody said or did in the past. While many people may hold non-medical models, which invoke the concepts of sin, karma, black magic, punishment, and supernatural causation, the biomedical disease model of psychosis should be presented. Providing information about a multifactorial etiology (brain pathology, genetic, and environmental factors) often helps in reducing feelings of distress, guilt, and blame among the relatives.

TABLE 8.2

Investigations to be Considered in the Assessment of Patients Presenting with Psychosis

- Electrolytes (for patients who are disoriented and in delirium)
- Erythrocyte sedimentation rate (to exclude chronic infections)
- Full blood examination
- Serum creatinine, blood sugar levels (if patient above 40 years of age)

In case of a doubt of organic illness, additional tests that need to be done include electroencephalogram (EEG) and cranial computed tomography (CT scan).

The importance of medication to control the symptoms should be emphasized. The relatives should be told that the symptoms may fluctuate over time and that medication can help by reducing current difficulties and preventing relapse.

Involvement in work and daily activities is important for recovery and rehabilitation. Relatives should also be helped to identify early signs of relapse and taught how to deal with it. Empowering patients and their families in the use of psychotropic medication will help them cope with fluctuations in symptoms and will not make them dependent on doctors. They should be taught how to manage sleep disturbance, restlessness, and early symptoms of psychotic relapse with the judicious use of antipsychotic medication.

Step 6. Prescribe medication

Antipsychotic medication will reduce psychotic symptoms. The dosage schedule and possible adverse effects (Table 8.3) must be discussed with the patient and family. The general principles of drug treatment include the use of the lowest possible dosage for the relief of symptoms, a gradual increase in doses in the elderly and close monitoring for side-effects. Smaller doses are generally required for psychosis secondary to medical conditions than for functional psychosis.

In addition to antipsychotic medication, benzodiazepines may be required to reduce agitation or assist with sleep, but they must be used only for a short period as they can produce dependence if used over a longer time. Anticholinergic drugs may be required to reduce antipsychotic-induced side-effects, which are common with older/typical antipsychotics and can be given prophylactically to prevent acute dystonia.

In general, after a single episode of psychosis, medication must be continued for 18–24 months. In case of a relapse or in chronic psychosis, the medication must be continued for longer periods. People with multiple episodes of illness with alternating phases of mania and depression require prophylaxis with mood stabilizers (e.g. lithium, sodium valproate, and carbamazepine; *see also* Chapter 23). They may require specialist input for their management.

Step 7. Discuss the role of psychosocial factors

Educate the family about the need for the patient to be supervised. Excessive stress and stimulation need to be reduced. It is not useful to argue with the patient's beliefs, though they may be wrong. Avoid confrontation unless it is necessary to prevent harmful or disruptive behavior.

Encourage the patient to maintain his or her daily routine of activities. Break chores into smaller steps. Offering rewards and praise, even if tasks are not perfectly done, will help to maintain and increase such behavior. Encourage re-entry into work when possible. It is also important to ensure that excessive demands are not made of the patient, as this could be detrimental to progress and may precipitate a relapse.

Offer patients health promotion and prevention measures, such as in the area of smoking cessation, weight control, exercise, diet, screening for diabetes, and sexual health.

TABLE 8.3

Common Antipsychotic Medications, their Side-effects, Indications, Dosage in Primary Care, and Duration of Treatment

Medication	Starting dose	Adult dose	Common side-effects	Indications	Duration of treatment
Non-sedating newer antipsychotics					
Risperidone	1–2 mg	2–6 mg	Extra-pyramidal symptoms, akathisia, sexual dysfunction, tardive dyskinesia	Conditions without marked agitation	At least 2 years after a first episode
Sedating newer antipsychotics					Needs to be continued for many years if there is a recurrence or a relapse of symptoms on withdrawal of drug
Olanzapine	5 mg	10–15 mg	Sedation, weight gain, elevation of blood sugar levels and lipids in predisposed, akathisia, tardive dyskinesia	Conditions associated with marked agitation, disturbed sleep	
Non-sedating older antipsychotics					
Haloperidol (oral or injection)	5 mg	5–10 mg	Extra-pyramidal symptoms, dystonia, akathisia, tardive dyskinesia	Given as intramuscular injection for severely disturbed; can be combined with injection promethazine, 25–50 mg IM, for greater sedation	
Other medication					
Lorazepam	1–2 mg	4–6 mg	Sedation, falls in elderly	Extreme agitation, restlessness	Gradually taper within 1–2 weeks
Trihexyphenidyl	2 mg	4–6 mg	Dry mouth, constipation, urinary retention, confusion	Extra-pyramidal symptoms (common with the use of older antipsychotics or high dose of the newer drugs)	Attempt withdrawal after 3–4 months without symptoms

TABLE 8.3

Common Antipsychotic Medications, their Side-effects, Indications, Dosage in Primary Care, and Duration of Treatment

Medication	Starting dose	Adult dose	Common side-effects	Indications	Duration of treatment
Promethazine hydrochloride (injection)	25 mg	25–50 mg	Sedation	For dystonia; or along with haloperidol for extreme disturbance	Single dose, intramuscular

Medication	Starting dose	Adult dose	Common side-effects	Indications	Optimal serum levels	Monitor
Lithium SR	400 mg	800–1200 mg	Tremors, diarrhoea, exacerbation of psoriasis, hypothyroidism, nephrotoxicity	Mania, hypomania; prophylaxis in bipolar disorder	0.6–1.0 mEq/L (plasma level to be checked 7 days after reaching a steady dose)	ECG, thyroid function tests, renal function tests to be done before starting lithium

Creatinine, TSH and serum lithium every 6–12 months |
| Carbamazepine plain or CR | 200 mg | 600–800 mg | Drowsiness, ataxia, nausea, generalized rash, low white cell count | Mania, hypomania; prophylaxis in bipolar disorder | 7–10 mg/L (plasma level to be checked 7 days after reaching a steady dose) | Liver function tests and blood counts prior to starting drug and every 6–12 months |
| Sodium valproate plain or CR | 200 mg | 800–1000 mg | Gastric irritation, lethargy, weight gain, hair loss | Mania, hypomania; prophylaxis in bipolar disorder | Titrate by effect and tolerability. Maintain between 50 and 150 mg/L | Liver function tests prior to starting drug and every 6–12 months |

BOX 8.2 CHRONIC PSYCHOSIS

A 22-year-old man was brought to the hospital by his parents, who reported that while his early development was normal, over the past few years it had been noticed that he kept to himself and had few friends. During the past year, he began to miss classes in college and his grades began to fall steadily. He began neglecting his personal care, rarely left his room, answered questions with few words and rarely expressed any emotions. His parents noticed that he occasionally muttered to himself. On examination of his mental status, he reported hearing multiple voices speaking to him even in the absence of people; these were commenting on his actions. He showed no emotional reactivity and his speech was minimal and difficult to follow. He did not report substance use, and his physical examination and routine laboratory investigations were within normal limits.

The antipsychotic medication risperidone was prescribed, beginning with 1 mg at night. This was gradually increased to 6 mg over 2 weeks. The anticholinergic agent trihexyphenidyl (2 mg) was added in the morning when the risperidone dose crossed 4 mg to prevent extrapyramidal symptoms. The patient was encouraged to remain active and carry out his daily activities. Compliance with medication was emphasized and regular appointments for review were given.

Step 8. Elaborate coping strategies

Family members need to be supported as they often have to cope unaided with the unpredictable and socially awkward behavior or persisting under-activity of their loved ones. Psychotic patients, especially those with chronic illness, often require sustained care, patience, and tolerance of their lack of insight regarding their own problems. This places a huge burden on the caregivers. Other stressors include coping with disturbed or violent behavior and concerns about the fate of adult children with chronic psychosis as they, the parents, age and are unable to provide care in the long term.

Reassure the relatives that recovery often takes place in small steps. Help them to remain optimistic, and emphasize the patient's strengths and abilities rather than deficits. In addition to providing support themselves, general practitioners may assist patients and relatives by encouraging them to benefit from the services provided by support organizations that may be available.

Step 9. Negotiate a treatment plan, compliance, participation, and responsibility

Untreated psychosis can result in harm to the patient by suicide and other forms of self-harm, deterioration of physical health due to neglect, and an overall decline in functioning. The possibility of harm to others under the influence of delusions and hallucinations is also possible. Many people with chronic mental illness can lead productive and fulfilling lives with appropriate treatment. Though the long-term prognosis may be difficult to predict, acute psychotic episodes often have a good

BOX 8.3   EPISODIC PSYCHOSIS

A 32-year-old man was brought to the hospital with a six-month history of being very suspicious that people were trying to harm him by poisoning his food, and that they were following him with cameras wherever he went. He believed that God was talking to him through the television and said he could hear voices of famous people commanding him to do various things. He was irritable and occasionally assaulted his relatives when they opposed him. He was seen laughing and talking to himself even when alone. He had stopped going to work, did not care for himself, and slept and ate poorly. The family reported that 3 years earlier he had had similar problems, for which he had been treated. He had improved after 8–10 months. Since then he had been reasonably well till the past six months. On examination of his mental status, he reported multiple auditory hallucinations, saying he heard politicians and celebrities speaking to him. He believed God was conveying messages to him through the television and had delusions that people were trying to harm him. He was animated when describing these, but was irritable if his views were challenged.

The sedative antipsychotic medication olanzapine was started at 5 mg at bedtime and the dose increased to 15 mg over a week. The relatives were advised not to challenge or confront the patient about his beliefs. The patient was encouraged to carry out his daily activities. Compliance with medication and regular follow-up were emphasized. He was maintained on antipsychotic prophylaxis to prevent future episodes.

prognosis. In substance-induced psychotic states, the symptoms generally last for hours, days or, at most, a few weeks after discontinuation of the substance.

Engage the caregivers collaboratively in the treatment process. Emphasize the need for regular, supervised medication. Simplify the medication regimen as much as possible to enhance compliance.

A focus on patient- and family-led plans, which focus on empowerment, hope, acceptance, and support, called the recovery model, is useful. Such a strategy will allow for meaning in people's lives and will reduce the emphasis on treatment-resistant symptoms and residual deficits.

Step 10. Give a specific appointment for review

Regular review of progress is necessary for all patients. There should be scheduled appointments every few days for acute psychosis and follow-up every 2–4 weeks. Monthly or even three-monthly reviews for people with psychosis who are stabilized will be needed. Periodic check-ups will also help to monitor compliance with medication, observe for and manage any adverse effects that may occur, and support and guide relatives.

BOX 8.4   ACUTE PSYCHOSIS

A 25-year-old student was brought to the hospital with a three-week history of abnormal behavior, which began after staying up over several nights while preparing for her examinations. She was noticed to be very talkative and very familiar even with people she did not know. She was hyperactive and very generous with her money, unlike her usual behavior. She was very cheerful, and confidently told everyone that she had become the "greatest thinker in the world" and had made several scientific discoveries in the 1 month that would ensure world peace. Her mother reported that a year back she had had a similar episode, from which she had recovered after treatment for a month. She was functioning well between episodes. On examination, her speech was rapid and difficult to interrupt. She quickly skipped from one idea to another and said that thoughts were racing through her mind. She had delusions that she had made great scientific discoveries but was unable to describe them. She appeared unusually cheerful and had an exaggerated sense of confidence.

The sedative antipsychotic medication olanzapine was started at 5 mg at bedtime and the dose increased to 15 mg over a week. The relatives were advised not to challenge and confront the patient about her beliefs. The patient was encouraged to carry out her daily activities. Compliance with medication and regular follow-up were emphasized. She was maintained on the mood stabilizer lithium as prophylaxis to prevent future episodes.

BOX 8.5   RECOVERY MODEL

Despite major advances in the treatment of severe mental illness, many people with major mental disorders continue to have disabling symptoms, incapacitating adverse medication effects, unresolved livelihood issues, and poor quality of life. In addition, the promise of the biomedical revolution has failed to help many people get back to their premorbid functioning and restore their employment and careers. Consequently, many patients, their families, and caregivers and mental health activists have argued that the continued focus on symptoms and medication in people with treatment resistant conditions, is less than optimal. They have proposed an alternative model of care called the "recovery model".

The recovery process should provide a holistic view of people with mental illness that focuses on the person, not just their symptoms. The recovery model argues that such recovery is possible and that it is a journey rather than a destination. It does not necessarily imply a return to premorbid level of functioning and asymptomatic phase of the person's life. Nor does it suggest a linear progression to recovery but one, which may happen in "fits and starts" and, like life, have many "ups and downs".

The recovery process is profoundly influenced by people's expectations and attitudes, and requires a well-organized system of support from family, friends, or professionals. The model calls for optimism and commitment from people with mental illness, their families, mental health professionals, public health teams, social services, and the community. It also requires the mental health system, primary care, public health, and social services to embrace new and innovative ways of working.

The recovery model aims to help people with mental illnesses and distress to look beyond mere survival and existence. It encourages them to move forward and set new goals. It supports the view that they should get on with their lives, do things, and develop relationships that give their lives meaning.

The model emphasizes that, while people may not have full control over their symptoms, they can have control over their lives. Recovery is not about "getting rid" of problems but seeing beyond a person's mental health problems, recognizing and fostering their abilities, interests, and dreams. It argues against the traditional concepts of mental illness and social attitudes, which often impose limits on people experiencing mental ill health. Health professionals often have reduced expectations, while families and friends can be overly protective or pessimistic about what someone with a mental health problem will be able to do and achieve. Recovery is about looking beyond those limits to help people achieve their own goals, aspirations, and dreams. Recovery can be a voyage of self-discovery and personal growth; experiences of mental illness can provide opportunities for change, and reflection and discovery of new values, skills, and interests.

Factors that supports recovery
Many factors are associated with the road to recovery and include good relationships, financial security, and satisfying work. The environment, which provides for personal growth, developing resilience to stress and adversity, and allows people to develop cultural and spiritual perspectives, is also crucial. Being believed in, listened to and understood by families, friends and health, and social service personnel are very helpful to people on the road to recovery. Getting explanations for problems or experiences and developing skills and receive support to achieve their goals are crucial to success. Support during periods of crisis is also critical.

Recovery and community
Many people with severe mental illness now live in the community. The closure of asylums and long stay psychiatric facilities has increased their numbers. And yet,

far too many people live isolated lives. Many psychiatric, community, and public health services fail to empower their users by engaging local neighborhoods and living in partnership with communities. Such active engagement and symbiotic relationship within community requires a mutual appreciation of the potential of people with and without mental health problems. The process of engagement and consequent recovery is strongly linked to social inclusion. A key role for mental health and social services is to support people to regain their place in the communities, take part in mainstream activities, and utilize opportunities for growth along with everyone else. There is growing evidence that supports the contention that taking part in social, educational, training, volunteering, and employment opportunities can support the process of individual recovery.

People with severe mental illness need to be supported to create their own recovery plans, set their own goals, map their processes, identify their strengths and weaknesses, recognize the road blocks, and facilitate good practice, which keeps them well.

WHEN SHOULD A PATIENT BE REFERRED FOR SPECIALIST HELP?

Referral to specialists should be considered as an emergency when the patient is at risk of harming himself or others due to suicide, violence, or neglect. It may also be required if there is a relapse, for multiple episodes of illness, refusal to take medication, lack of response to prescribed medication, problematic side-effects or concerns about comorbid drug or alcohol use.

CONCLUSION

Recognizing the symptoms, ensuring the safety of patients and their relatives, initiating antipsychotic medication, psychosocial management, providing support, and empowering patients and the families are necessary components of the treatment package for subjects with psychosis.

9 Physical Symptoms, Health Anxiety, and Common Mental Disorders

Many patients, with psychosocial and psychiatric problems, present to general medical settings with persistent worries about their health. Such patients can present with medically unexplained symptoms and/or excessive concerns about their health. They may often have associated symptoms of depression and anxiety. Such presentations are also frequently associated with psychosocial stress, stressful life events, poor coping, and limited social support. The sub-categorization into different disorders such as depression, anxiety, somatoform disorders, and hypochondriasis is difficult because of milder symptoms, sub-syndromal and mixed presentations.

Their management includes the exclusion of medical and organic causes and symptomatic management. Antidepressants can be used for those with anxiety, depression, and persistent pain. Psychosocial management, crucial for success, includes the acknowledgment of distress, elicitation of patient perspectives, education about the nature of the illness, identification of coexistent stress, a discussion of general and specific coping strategies, negotiating a treatment plan, and review.

INTRODUCTION

Family physicians and general practitioners (GPs) often encounter patients with persistent symptoms and concerns about health. Such patients repeatedly seek medical attention despite failure to detect abnormalities on physical examinations, normal laboratory parameters, and professional reassurance regarding the absence of major medical disease. They usually report distressing physical symptoms for which known medical causes are not found. Such patients often have emotional and psychosocial problems. These clinical presentations include a diverse range of patterns including:

1. *Medically Unexplained Symptoms:* This label has been considered inappropriate as it overemphasizes the centrality of medically unexplained symptoms, grounds a diagnosis on the absence of a medical explanation, reinforces mind–body dualism, and is pejorative, demeaning, and implies that the symptoms are not "real".
2. *Specific Physical Symptoms* without specific medical cause (e.g. headache, specific symptom labels used by GPs to focus on the reason for the clinical encounter;

somatic symptom disorder, a term now used by psychiatrists for people with somatic symptoms and associated excessive anxiety and concerns about health).

3. *Medical Conditions* with fluctuation with psychosocial stress (e.g. irritable bowel syndrome, non-cardiac chest pain).
4. *Illness Anxiety and Hypochondriasis* are defined as presentations without/mild somatic symptoms but with excessive preoccupation and anxiety about having a serious illness.
5. *Anxiety, Depression, and Common Mental Disorders*, which can present with somatic symptoms.

Such presentations are common in primary and secondary care, associated with disability and poorer quality of life and they result in frequent visits to medical practitioner and hospitals. This chapter discusses a simple approach to managing such patients in primary care and in general medical settings.

WHAT IS HEALTH ANXIETY?

Health anxiety is a label used to describe clinical presentations of people with or without somatic symptoms and who may or may not have diagnosable medical diseases, who present with a preoccupation about having or acquiring and a serious illness. They have a high level of anxiety about their health, are easily alarmed about their personal health status and frequently seek medical examination, intervention, and reassurance.

Such presentations are common with the increase in medicalization of distress in society. The breakdown of traditional family, social and community supports, and the increase in the use of the internet make anxious people to selectively focus on the most serious explanation for symptoms, even though these may be very uncommon. Such anxiety is often disabling and is associated with long-term morbidity and increased sick leave and absence from work.

WHAT ARE COMMON MENTAL DISORDERS?

The term common mental disorder is used to describe psychiatric presentations typically encountered in the community and in primary care. These patients usually present with physical complaints, which do not have a medical cause, significant anxiety regarding their health and other symptoms of anxiety and depression. These presentations are milder, mixed, and frequently associated with psychosocial adversity, differentiating these disorders from those that present to psychiatric settings. The first stop for people with such psychiatric conditions is often the GP. Common psychiatric conditions seen in primary care include anxiety, depression, phobia, panic, obsessive–compulsive disorder, health anxiety, and problems secondary to acute and chronic stress (Table 9.1).

HOW COMMON ARE PSYCHIATRIC SYNDROMES IN PRIMARY CARE?

Most reports of the prevalence of psychiatric problems in primary care and general medical settings have documented that one-third to one-fourth of patients have a diagnosable psychiatric disorder.

TABLE 9.1

A Brief Description of Common Psychiatric Presentations and Labels

Anxiety: The apprehensive anticipation of future danger or misfortune, accompanied by feelings of dysphoria or somatic symptoms of tension. The focus of the anticipated danger may be internal or external.

Depression: Persistent sadness, low mood, and loss of interest or pleasure in nearly all activities. It is often associated with sleep disturbance, loss of appetite and weight, decreased libido, and suicidal ideation.

Obsessive–compulsive disorder: The presence of recurrent obsessions (persistent ideas, thoughts, impulses, or images which are experienced as intrusive and inappropriate and cause marked anxiety or distress), or compulsions (repetitive behaviors or mental acts whose aim is to reduce anxiety). These are often time-consuming, distressing, and cause significant impairment in functioning. The patients can appreciate the irrational nature of the obsessions and compulsions.

Panic: The sudden onset of intense apprehension, fearfulness, and terror, often associated with a feeling of impending doom. These episodes last for a short duration (less than 30 minutes) and may be associated with anticipatory anxiety and phobic avoidance.

Phobia: A persistent, irrational fear of a specific object or situation. This often leads either to avoidance of the stimulus or situation, or to enduring it with dread.

WHAT ARE THE COMMON CLINICAL PRESENTATIONS OF PSYCHIATRIC AND PSYCHOSOCIAL PROBLEMS SEEN IN PRIMARY CARE AND GENERAL HOSPITAL SETTINGS?

The most common clinical presentations of psychiatric problems are that of physical symptoms and anxiety regarding health. The general population expects doctors to manage physical complaints rather than psychological and social distress. In addition, psychiatric disorders have many somatic and physical symptoms. Consequently, patients presenting to general medical settings with psychiatric and psychosocial problems often report somatic complaints. On the other hand, some people with health anxiety are so concerned that they may have a feared diagnosis that they avoid consultations with physicians.

WHAT HAPPENS TO PATIENTS WHO DO NOT GET HELP FROM PHYSICIANS?

The inability of physicians to identify physical causes for somatic symptoms and manage such presentations often results in the physician downplaying their importance and ignoring the patient's distress. Consequently, many patients are often discontented with the medical consultation and the care and treatment that they receive. Such dissatisfaction results in many patients visiting other doctors and hospitals, shopping for different treatments and solutions.

WILL SUCH PATIENTS PRESENT WITH PSYCHOLOGICAL SYMPTOMS LIKE THOSE OF ANXIETY AND DEPRESSION?

Yes, they may have such symptoms. However, most patients will mention these mental symptoms only on detailed enquiry. Most focus on their health and somatic symptoms, placing reduced emphasis on mental distress. While they may often recognize the association of physical and mental symptoms to psychosocial distress, they frequently expect tablets and medication to relieve them of their suffering.

WILL I BE ABLE TO DIAGNOSE ANXIETY, DEPRESSION AND OTHER PSYCHIATRIC SYNDROMES?

While patients may report these symptoms, it is often difficult to differentiate these syndromes in patients who present to primary care. Anxiety and depression share many symptoms, such as weakness, tiredness, fatigue, lethargy, difficulty in concentration, sleep disturbance, and worry. The typical symptoms of anxiety and of depression are commonly seen in the same patient. These symptoms are often mild, which makes the differentiation of the two classical syndromes very difficult. This also applies to other syndromes such as phobia, panic and obsessive–compulsive disorder. However, one does occasionally see classical psychiatric syndromes in primary care. The general protocol will allow you to manage these patients without making a particular psychiatric diagnosis. The protocol is simple and flexible to allow specific and additional treatments, which you may consider appropriate.

BOX 9.1 PHYSICAL SYMPTOMS AND PERSONAL FEARS

A 30-year-old married woman presented with chest discomfort, multiple aches and pains, fatigue, and a lack of concentration. She denied symptoms of depression, anxiety, and stress. However, on enquiry she mentioned that she had two children and did not want any more. She admitted that her husband and she were not practicing contraception. Her physical examination and routine laboratory investigation were within normal limits.

She was educated about the nature of her symptoms. The distress was acknowledged, but the focus was on the absence of disease and the need for contraception. She was also prescribed vitamin tablets.

BOX 9.2 PHYSICAL SYMPTOMS AND MARITAL DISCORD

A 40-year-old married woman presented with headache, aches and pains, weakness, fatigue, and sleep disturbance. She appeared sad during the interview. On enquiry, she mentioned that her husband had an alcohol problem and physically assaulted her regularly. Her physical examination and routine laboratory investigations were within normal limits.

She was educated about the nature of her symptoms. The distress was acknowledged, but the focus was on the absence of disease and on the need to resolve the marital discord and help her husband quit the habit. She was empowered by discussing the different options available to her, including talking to her parents, her in-laws, the village elders, and the police. She was prescribed a small dose of a sedative antidepressant.

WILL I BE ABLE TO MANAGE SUCH PATIENTS WITHOUT REACHING A SPECIFIC DIAGNOSIS?

Yes, you will be able to treat such patients. All these syndromes usually require psychological and social support and counseling. People with severe distress and disability may also need antidepressant medication. The steps to deliver these are mentioned in this chapter. The protocol contains all the essential steps in the management of these conditions.

WHAT IS THE BASIS OF THE SUGGESTED PROTOCOL?

The "10-step" approach described is based on the "reattribution model". This method has been developed in collaboration with GPs over many years and modified over time to incorporate important psychiatric and physician principles. The steps, the sequence, and their rationale are briefly described.

WHAT ARE THE TEN STEPS?

The ten steps in management are:

1. Recognize the clinical presentation
2. Acknowledge distress
3. Elicit the patient's and the family's perspective
4. Take a focused history; carry out physical examination and laboratory investigations to rule out medical problems
5. Educate the patient about the nature of illness and its treatment
6. Prescribe medication
7. Discuss the role of stress as cause and consequence of illness

---

BOX 9.3 CHEST PAIN AND FREQUENT VISITS TO EMERGENCY DEPARTMENT

A 50-year old man frequently presented to the emergency department of the hospital with sudden episodes of palpitations, sweating, tremor, giddiness, and chest pain. He felt that he was going to die. These attacks lasted 10–15 minutes and seemed to resolve spontaneously but left him anxious and distressed. These attacks had made him housebound. Detailed history did not suggest exertion dyspnea or chest pain induced by effort. Despite repeated investigations including ECG, ECHO, and evaluation of enzymes, being within normal limits, he was fearful that he might die of a heart attack.

A patient enquiry into his fears revealed that his uncle had died of a myocardial infarction and he had read that it ran in families. He was counseled about the absence of physical disease, psychological nature of his symptoms, the need to recognize and change thought patterns and behavior, which triggered panic and anxiety. He was taught relaxation exercises, breathing retraining, and positive visualization. He was advised to learn yoga and meditation. He was also prescribed a selective serotonin uptake inhibitor.

8. Elaborate coping strategies
9. Negotiate a treatment plan, compliance, participation and responsibility
10. Give an appointment for review.

Step 1. Recognize the clinical presentation

Patients with common psychiatric problems often present to primary care. These problems include psychosocial problems, which result in non-psychotic disorders. They may present with physical symptoms or with excessive worry about their health. They

---

BOX 9.4 SEXUAL CONCERNS

A 20-year-old man presented with recurrent aches and pains, tiredness and fatigue. His physical examination was within normal limits as were his basic laboratory investigations. Open-ended questioning about his circumstances revealed that his symptoms coincided with the fact that he had started dating. He did admit that he was anxious about sex and that he occasionally reported premature ejaculation. Detailed enquiry revealed that he was stressed at work and that he had recently changed jobs, moved to another city, and that he met his girlfriend once a month.

Elicitation of his sexual concerns followed by explanation of sexual function and the fact that it was normal to have occasional premature ejaculation, especially when sex was not frequent, was reassuring. His symptoms gradually remitted as he regained his confidence.

BOX 9.5 CLEANLINESS CONCERNS

A 30-year-old man presented to his GP with headache, of 6 months' duration. Enquiry into his complaints revealed that his symptom coincided with an increase in his concerns related to cleanliness. He was always a neat person, who liked to keep everything in place. He would wash his hands after work but did not fuss about it. He noticed that for the past year he started getting the urge to repeatedly wash his hands as he felt that he might have contacted some infection. Gradually the time for washing had increased and he now spent over half an hour on each occasion. These rituals had made him housebound. He realized that his thoughts and action were not rational but he became distressed if he did not give into his urge to repeatedly wash his hands. He was embarrassed about his symptoms.

He was diagnosed to have obsessive–compulsive disorder and was started on fluoxetine. He was advised counseling. The irrational basis of his fears, its detrimental impact on his mental health, rationale to change his behavior, and the need to reduce the time for washing was discussed. With the support of his therapist, he was gradually able to reduce the time taken to wash his hands.

can also have symptoms of anxiety, depression, phobia, panic, obsessive–compulsive disorder, and adjustment problems secondary to acute and chronic stress. While very few patients complain of psychological distress, the majority usually report distressing physical symptoms for which known medical causes are not found or excessive anxiety and a preoccupation regarding their health even in the absence of physical symptoms. These concerns do not respond to medical reassurance or negative diagnostic tests. Anxiety about illness takes a prominent place in the individual's life and becomes a characteristic response to stressful events.

Other common clinical presentations, which need to be excluded, are disorientation (delirium), chronic memory loss (dementia), substance dependence, and strange beliefs, hallucinations, and grossly abnormal behavior (psychosis).

Step 2. Acknowledge distress

Acknowledging the distress caused by the physical symptoms reassures the patient that his symptoms will be carefully considered rather than dismissed. The failure to do so is often interpreted by patients as an indication that the physician has not understood the problem or that he/she does not believe the symptoms to be genuine. Acknowledging distress reflects an empathetic attitude, and contributes to the establishment of an effective rapport and the formation of a therapeutic alliance, which are essential in facilitating improvement.

Step 3. Elicit the patient's and the family's perspective on symptoms

Providing appropriate reassurance is an important part of the medical consultation. It is most effective if based on the patient's actual concerns. Asking patients what they think or fear is wrong with them is useful in addressing specific concerns (e.g. "It could be cancer").

Many beliefs held by patients with unexplained physical symptoms contradict the biomedical model of their illness. They may hold strong beliefs related to the fact that they actually have physical disease even in the absence of clinical and laboratory evidence, on the one hand, while having doubts about the possibility of a medical disorder, on the other. They may also hold multiple beliefs about their condition, which incorporate supernatural causation (e.g. karma, sin, black magic, punishment, etc.), or subscribe to local cultural explanations that poor diet and nutrition, excessive work, and poverty are causal.

The patient's beliefs need to be discussed before presenting alternative biomedical explanations. Outright rejection of the patient's beliefs about his illness early in the consultation or a failure to elicit his beliefs often proves disastrous. Eliciting such explanations will also allow for focused examination, investigations, and specific reassurance.

Step 4. Take a focused history; carry out physical examination and laboratory investigations

Physical disease, substance dependence, and psychosis (e.g. presence of strange beliefs, hallucinations, and grossly abnormal behavior) have to be excluded. A focused history,

BOX 9.6   DIFFERENT APPROACHES TO COMMON MENTAL DISORDERS

The approach of GPs and family physicians differs from that adopted by psychiatrists. Differences in practice settings, population served, and medical perspectives between psychiatrists and primary healthcare professionals are responsible for the differences in approach. GPs see people with milder, non-specific symptoms, sub-syndromal, and mixed presentations. These presentations often clustering around the "case severity threshold" and are frequently associated with psychosocial adversity. Consequently, primary care physicians prefer categories such as mixed anxiety depressive disorder and adjustment disorders to conventional psychiatric diagnosis (e.g. depressive disorder and generalized anxiety disorder as separate diseases). However, mixed anxiety and depression and adjustment reactions are not included in the standard psychiatric classifications, even for use in primary care. These categories do not find a place in standard psychiatric guidelines for use in general practice (e.g. the mhGAP diagnostic and management guideline). Categories useful in primary care seem to be unacceptable to specialists and unsuitable in their settings and vice versa.

The lower prevalence in traditional psychiatric diagnosis (e.g. generalized anxiety and depressive disorder) result in high false-positive rates, as predictive values are prevalence dependent. Family physicians argue that many patients diagnosed with major depression/depressive episode often have concurrent psychosocial adversity have high rates of spontaneous remission and of placebo response and those with mild-to-moderate severity do not respond to antidepressants.

Family physicians place a great deal of emphasis on the presence and impact of psychosocial circumstances (e.g. stress, personal resources, coping, social supports, and culture) on mental health. They are reluctant to use symptom counts, sans context, to label people. They argue that psychiatric labels identify those in distress than those with disease. GPs also understand local contexts and are able to recognize and acknowledge multiple variants of emotional distress. These realities force GPs to favor the recording of reasons for the clinical encounter or the recognition of broader clinical presentations rather than use specific psychiatric labels.

A serious concern raised by family physicians is the medicalization of human distress. Physicians seem to be uncomfortable with the use of the concept of mental disorder, with its disease halo, which sidesteps the disease–illness dichotomy while encompassing both disease and distress. Consequently, GPs, family and primary care physicians use the International Classification of Primary Care-2 (ICPC-2), which focuses on reasons for clinical encounters, patient data and clinical activity. They argue that patients seek medical help when they are disturbed or distressed, when they are in pain or are worried about the implication of their symptoms. These forms of distress largely require emotional and social support.

physical examination, and laboratory investigation to exclude physical diseases are cardinal.

Recognizing the chronic nature of the many complaints without the presence of objective evidence of serious medical disease and feeding this information back to the patient is useful. A review of previous laboratory investigations and feedback on the patient's normalcy will add to the patient's confidence that physical disease has been excluded. The failure of the many symptomatic treatments to completely resolve the complaints is also a useful pointer that only medication-based strategies will not remove the symptoms unless stress and coping issues, which may underlie the distress, are sorted out.

Such brief yet systematic examination will go a long way in reassuring the patient that medical causes have not been overlooked. A cursory examination, on the other hand, makes the patient believe that a serious attempt was not made to rule out medical disease and leaves him dissatisfied with the consultation.

The extent of laboratory investigation, which should be done, is dependent on the clinical presentation. Basic tests may be required to identify conditions that do not have clinical signs and pathognomonic manifestations. Anemia can be ruled out by clinical examination. Total and differential white cell counts are useful in excluding tropical eosinophilia. The erythrocyte sedimentation rate (ESR) continues to be a useful investigation to exclude tuberculosis in the developing world; high ESR values should be investigated. Serum creatinine is useful in patients with hypertension. Blood sugar levels are necessary to rule out diabetes mellitus in people over 40 years of age and those with a family history. Lipid profiles and electrocardiogram is mandated in people over 40 years of age, especially those who present with possible cardiac symptoms.

Step 5. Educate the patient about the illness and treatment

Reassurance is crucial in allaying the patient's concern and changing their help-seeking behavior. A common expectation among patients is a better understanding of their symptoms. Being told that there is no serious medical problem underlying their symptoms is effective in reducing the health concern for many patients. However, for a significant number such reassurance alone is not helpful, resulting in further needless consultations. Evidence suggests that for reassurance to be effective, the patient's concerns need to be elicited; appropriate and alternative explanations provided. Worrying about their health is bound to recur if the symptoms persist, especially if the patients do not receive a satisfactory explanation that enables them to interpret their recurrent symptoms as benign. Consequently, it becomes necessary to manage the patient's beliefs, misconceptions, and concerns about health.

Explanations, which completely deny all diseases often, make patients wonder if the doctor disbelieves their symptoms. The emphasis should be on reassuring the patient about the absence of any serious physical disease while acknowledging the reality of and distress caused by the symptoms. The possibility of a catastrophic event or incapacitation being highly unlikely should be reiterated. Alternative explanations for these symptoms (i.e. the individual's tendency to interpret innocuous bodily sensations as bodily dysfunctions or thatsymptoms may be related to stress) are useful. Other explanations, such as recognizing that their body is structurally normal while being functionally different, are also useful in certain conditions (e.g. irritable bowel syndrome).

Discussing the link between physical symptoms and stress is crucial. Simple explanations of how anxiety and stress may cause physical symptoms or how depression lowers the threshold of pain are useful. Asking if anyone else in the family or among friends has suffered from similar symptoms also helps patients identify such mechanisms. These patients commonly report interpersonal problems, financial difficulties, alcohol dependence in the spouse and physical abuse, usually on enquiry. Other stressors, which also cause anxiety, include sexual misconceptions and dysfunction in men, and a fear of unwanted pregnancy in women who are not practicing contraception.

The emphasis should be on providing reassurance about the absence of physical disease while acknowledging the reality of and distress caused by the symptoms.

Step 6. Prescribe medication

Many patients expect medication. Patients who have the following conditions may benefit from antidepressant medication: moderate-to-severe distress, symptoms of severe anxiety and depression, and severe stress. Antidepressant medication can also be prescribed if panic, phobia, or obsessive–compulsive symptoms are identified. It is useful in conditions where pain is chronic and incapacitating (e.g. headache, irritable bowel syndrome, atypical chest pain).

The choice of antidepressant medication is based on whether the patient has insomnia or is sleeping well. Sedative antidepressants should be used in patients who have sleep disturbance. Such sedative medication includes tricyclics and mirtazapine (Table 9.2). The use of non-sedative selective serotonin reuptake inhibitors (SSRIs) in patients with insomnia will result in the use of benzodiazepines and the possibility of addiction.

Tricyclic antidepressants, such as dothiepin, imipramine, and amitriptyline (25–150 mg/day), are especially useful in patients with insomnia. The common side-effects include sedation, giddiness, dry mouth, and constipation. These antidepressants can result in cardiac conduction delays, especially in those with compromised cardiac functions. The patient should be started at the smallest dose possible and the dosage should be gradually increased every few days up to a dose, which is tolerated by the patient. Higher dosages may have incapacitating adverse effects and could result in poor compliance. Many benefit from smaller doses (25–75 mg per day).

Mirtazapine (7.5–15 mg/day) is a sedative antidepressant that does not have specific cardiac adverse effects. It is a newer antidepressant that can be considered in those with insomnia, but it is more expensive than tricyclic antidepressants. However, its adverse impact on plasma glucose makes it less suitable for those with diabetes and metabolic syndrome.

Selective serotonin reuptake inhibitors can be used in people with distress, depression, and persistent pain without sleep disturbance. Fluoxetine, sertraline and

TABLE 9.2

Common Medications, their Side-effects, Indications, Dosages, and Duration of Treatment

Medication	Starting dose	Adult dose	Common side-effects	Indications*	Duration of treatment
Dothiepin/ dosulepin, imipramine, amitriptyline	25 mg	50–150 mg	Sedation, giddiness, dry mouth, constipation	Conditions associated with disturbed sleep	3–6 months followed by a tapering schedule
Mirtazapine	7.5 mg	15 mg	Sedation	Conditions associated with disturbed sleep; cardiac disease	Can be continued for many years in case of relapse of symptoms on withdrawal
Fluoxetine	20 mg	20 mg	Nausea, abdominal discomfort, restlessness	Conditions without sleep disturbance	
Citalopram	20 mg	20 mg			
Sertraline	25 mg	50–100 mg			

*Indications include unexplained physical symptoms, depression, anxiety, panic, phobia, obsessive–compulsive disorder

citalopram are non-sedative and have fewer adverse effects than the tricyclic agents, though they can produce nausea and restlessness. Many such drugs have the same starting and maximum dosage for use in general medical practice.

In general, antidepressants are prescribed for 3–6 months, after which they are tapered. They can be continued for many years if a relapse of symptoms occurs on withdrawal. "Start low and go slow" is the principle in medication dosage. Lower doses and slower increases are necessary in children, in the elderly, and in patients with liver and kidney disease and dysfunction.

Patients without the symptoms described above can be given vitamins and the placebo response often helps them cope with their circumstances. Benzodiazepines are best avoided as they produce dependence, if prescribed for more than 1 month.

Step 7. Discuss the role of stress as cause and as consequence

Stress is commonly associated with medically unexplained symptoms, health anxiety, and with common mental disorders. Although recent psychiatric classifications discount the role of context and focus on symptom counts to arrive at a diagnosis, good clinicians are aware of the need to explore the context and understand the patient's situation and life. Stress can be causal or a consequence of such symptoms. Mentioning the possible link between stress and symptoms is usually a good introduction to eliciting the patient's personal circumstances and distress.

Men, especially in the younger age group, commonly present with physical symptoms when they have sexual misconceptions or dysfunction. Doubts about structure, function, and contraception may result in symptoms of fatigue and problems in concentration and memory. Premature ejaculation and erectile dysfunction can also cause medically unexplained symptoms. Sex, in many non-western cultures, is often not discussed in school and at home, and so information on the subject may be inaccurate or may exaggerate normal function, leading to feelings of inadequacy. A direct enquiry usually results in a detailed discussion on the subject. Specific education and treatment are helpful for sexual misconceptions, sexual dysfunction, and the lack of contraception.

Women who are sexually active and want to avoid pregnancy but do not use contraception are particularly prone to medically unexplained symptoms. The sick role usually exempts them from sex on many occasions, but the risk of pregnancy is ever-present. Simple contraceptive advice will often help to solve the problem.

The other commonly encountered stressors include interpersonal conflicts, marital discord, alcohol use by the spouse, domestic violence, financial difficulties, job-related stress, and problems with the children's education.

The identification of the possible link between stress and medically unexplained symptoms, anxiety and depression is necessary for the patient to realize the need for personal solutions. It also takes away the need to shop for medical treatments. Even if patients deny the presence of stress, a mention of the possible mechanisms commonly seen in such presentations will get them thinking. The doctor needs to discuss the fact that such stress is common and that patients should consider resolving the stress to relieve the symptoms.

Many physicians refuse to enter into such discussions for fear of not being able to help. The realization that the doctor's responsibility is not to solve all personal and social distress but to empower the patient to consider the different options is liberating. Often, life situations may be difficult to resolve and may require acceptance and a change in coping strategies. Other situations may have simple solutions, which the person has not considered. A discussion on the possible role of such stress is a usual start to the therapeutic relationship, which can later explore possible problem-solving strategies.

Step 8. Elaborate coping strategies

General psychological measures, such as yoga, meditation, regular physical exercise, involvement in religious activities, hobbies, and leisure, help to improve coping and are useful for those under stress. Such coping strategies should be incorporated into the patient's daily routine, rather than be reserved for weekends, to be beneficial. These strategies are useful for everyone, not just for those who are not able to cope with the stress of living.

While some forms of social adversity can be easily altered, many require a change in philosophy, attitude, and lifestyle. Patients with specific problems will need help with problem-solving. Asking patients to look for specific solutions to their difficulties and giving them the time to examine the issues is obligatory. Coping will need to be discussed in subsequent consultations.

Step 9. Negotiate a treatment plan

Most patients expect cures from doctors and come back with the same or new complaints for the physician to resolve. The responsibility for improvement should be gently but firmly transferred to the patient. The offer of psychological support will help patients cope with stress. Compliance with the treatment regimen is crucial, as is patient participation in stress reduction programs and in improving coping strategies.

Step 10. Give a specific appointment for review

Regular review of progress is necessary for most patients. There should be scheduled, brief appointments every 2–4 weeks (i.e. avoiding "as-needed" appointments). A brief, focused physical examination must be performed at each visit to help rule out any new or worrisome condition and provide the patient with the important benefits of "laying on of hands". The physician should gradually shift the focus away from the patient's physical symptoms to the psychosocial context that may be most affecting him/her. The restoration of function rather than complete elimination of symptoms must be the goal of treatment. Most patients will accept this when they realize that their life circumstances are the cause of their symptoms. These visits can be used to provide psychological support and to discuss alternative coping strategies.

WILL I BE ABLE TO DO THIS IN MY BUSY CLINICAL PRACTICE?

Yes, physicians often worry that managing psychosocial problems takes time. With practice, the efficiency of the technique used improves and such counseling can be used in real-life situations. Even long interviews do not usually last more than 10–15 minutes.

WILL I BE ABLE TO SOLVE THE PATIENT'S PSYCHOSOCIAL PROBLEM?

Physicians often hesitate to get involved because of the fear that they will not be able to solve the patient's troubles. It is important to realize that the physician's responsibility is not to solve the patient's social difficulty but to empower patients to resolve it themselves. The specific solution to social adversity has to be the patient's own.

HOW CAN I BECOME SKILLED AT SUCH TREATMENT?

While the knowledge of the treatment process can be easily assimilated, the mastery of the skills required to manage such patients need rehearsal. With regular practice, it is possible to acquire competence and confidence in one's ability to handle patients with such presentations. Mastery of the technique increases the satisfaction that one derives from the process.

WHEN SHOULD I REFER A PATIENT FOR SPECIALIST HELP?

Referral to specialists should be avoided as these patients are best managed in primary care settings. Psychiatric evaluation and specialist counseling may be necessary for incapacitating mental disorders, intractable interpersonal difficulties, persistent sexual dysfunction, and chronic substance dependence.

CONCLUSION

Acknowledging the distress caused by symptoms, reassuring patients about the absence of serious physical illness, exploring and managing stress, and recognizing and treating distressing symptoms are necessary components of management packages for subjects with unexplained physical symptoms. Providing alternative explanations for the symptoms within the supportive context of a doctor–patient relationship and encouraging patients to pursue alternative coping strategies will help change knowledge and attitudes related to the illness and consequent practice.

Section III

Other Specific Presentations

10 Attempted Suicide and Suicide Risk

Patients at risk for suicide and those who harm themselves and attempt suicide are frequently brought to hospitals for help and treatment. The assessment includes the evaluation of the circumstances, stress, planning, and method employed. The examination of potential factors, which increase the risk of suicide (older age, male sex, single status, physical illness, and poor social support), severe depression, and psychosis is mandatory. The medical consequences of the suicidal attempt will have to be managed.

Acknowledging distress, elicitation of patient perspectives, understanding the context and stress, provision of support and education, discussion of general and specific measures of coping, negotiating a treatment plan, and regular review and follow-up are necessary. Psychotropic medication, psychiatric referral, and hospitalization are required for those with persistent and high risk.

INTRODUCTION

A minority of patients who attempt self-harm are admitted for psychiatric care. Many remain in the community. Many are brought to hospital after an attempt of deliberate self-harm. A majority of people who ultimately commit suicide seem to visit their physicians before the attempt. Consequently, physicians are in a position to effectively assess a person's needs by asking his patients about suicidal thoughts and feelings, identifying problems that may lead to such emotions, managing distress, and initiating appropriate care so as to prevent self-harm. This chapter discusses a simple approach to managing such patients in primary care.

WHAT ARE THE COMMON REASONS FOR SUICIDAL IDEATION?

Suicide is an event that is contributed to by a variety of factors. One of the most common is the distress a person experiences because of various problems in his or her life. These may include conflicts within the family – with the spouse, in-laws, parents or children, sexual conflicts and problematic relationships, financial hardship, failure in examinations and in love, difficulties at the workplace, humiliation, and shame. These problems may be acute or may be long-standing and chronic.

WHAT ARE THE OTHER COMMON CONTRIBUTORS TO SUICIDAL IDEATION?

The presence of a psychiatric illness, substance use disorders, severe medical illnesses (such as cancer, head injury, peptic ulcer disease, HIV/AIDS, and chronic pain), and an individual's personality structure are some of the other factors that result in suicidal ideation. Domestic violence and marital discord, lack of confiding relationships, and social supports are also contributory.

WHAT ARE THE COMMON PSYCHIATRIC DISORDERS THAT CAN RESULT IN SUICIDAL IDEATION?

The most common psychiatric conditions seen in primary care that can lead to suicidal ideation include depression, psychosis, personality disorders, and substance abuse problems. The presence of a psychiatric disorder increases a person's risk of attempting suicide.

WHICH ARE THE GROUPS AT A GREATER RISK FOR SUICIDE?

Adolescents, young adults, and the elderly have the highest suicide rates. Among the elderly, men are more likely than women to commit suicide; however, among the other age groups there are no marked differences between men and women. The other risk factors include previous suicide attempts and a family history of suicide or psychiatric illness. Those who are single, separated, widowed, or divorced, particularly if they live alone, run a greater risk of committing suicide.

HOW COMMONLY DO PEOPLE WITH SUICIDAL IDEATION PRESENT TO A PRIMARY CARE PHYSICIAN?

Most studies report that a majority of adults with suicidal ideation had visited a primary care physician within a few months before their attempt. The recognition and identification of suicidal thoughts is, therefore, an essential component of patient care.

Many physicians may be uncomfortable asking questions regarding self-harm and suicide for fear of upsetting the patient and her or his family. There are often concerns about "inducing" or encouraging such thoughts in one who does not have such ideas. In fact, most patients who have suicidal thoughts are ambivalent about those feelings and feel relieved at the chance to talk about such thoughts and ideas. Comprehensive assessment and intervention can save the patient's life.

HOW DO PATIENTS WHO ATTEND PRIMARY CARE MANIFEST THEIR SUICIDAL THOUGHTS?

Few patients in primary care report psychological distress; the majority present to general physicians and hospitals with medically unexplained physical symptoms. On specific questioning, symptoms such as weakness, tiredness, difficulty in concentration, sleep disturbance, or feelings of anxiety and sadness may be reported. Others may report anger, frustration, or distress over various stressors in their life. In such individuals, it is important to further enquire into their emotional state.

WHAT QUESTIONS DO I ASK TO ELICIT SUICIDAL THOUGHTS AND IDEAS?

During the initial evaluation of new patients, questions about a history of psychiatric disorders, substance abuse, and suicide attempts need to be included. Asking patients about how they feel emotionally, or about their mood, will encourage them to talk about their concerns. Patients who indicate a depressed or anxious mood or those who report recent or chronic stress should be asked, "Have things become so bad that you have considered taking your own life?" or "Sometimes when people feel sad or depressed or have problems in their lives they think about suicide. Have you ever thought about suicide?" If the patient admits to such thoughts, further questions are necessary. One should enquire about the duration and onset of suicidal ideation, plans ("Have you made any plans to harm yourself?"), the seriousness and dangerousness of the patient's intent, and the patient's access to harmful medications or other means of suicide.

WHAT HAPPENS TO PATIENTS WHO DO NOT GET HELP FROM PHYSICIANS?

Identifying such patients can help to understand their needs, offer assistance, and avert similar problems in the future. While there is no foolproof way of preventing suicide even with intervention, the risk of further attempts can be reduced.

WHAT ARE THE STEPS IN MANAGEMENT?

The ten steps in management are:

1. Recognize the clinical presentation
2. Acknowledge distress
3. Elicit the patient's and the family's perspective
4. Take a focused history; carry out physical examination and laboratory investigations to rule out medical problems
5. Educate the patient about the nature of illness and its treatment
6. Prescribe medication
7. Discuss the role of stress as cause and consequence of problems
8. Elaborate coping strategies
9. Negotiate a treatment plan, compliance, participation, and responsibility
10. Give an appointment for review.

Step 1. Recognize the clinical presentation and identify risk factors for suicide

Suicidal risk should be assessed in patients who have made a suicidal attempt or who are distressed about their circumstances in life. Based on the available details, it is important to establish a clinical judgment on the risk of suicide.

Demographic risk factors include the elderly, adolescent, and young adult groups, those who live alone, those with poor social supports, those with previous suicide attempts, and those with a family history of suicide. People with single marital status, separate, divorced, widowed, and recently bereaved are at higher risk. Those with chronic pain and physical illness are also susceptible.

Symptoms that increase the risk of suicide include hopelessness, agitation, and feelings of meaninglessness, poor self-esteem, and hallucinations. Psychiatric disorders that are commonly associated with suicide include depression, alcohol or drug abuse, bipolar disorders, schizophrenia and other psychotic disorders, and personality disorders.

Direct enquiry into whether the patient has experienced thoughts of suicide, or made plans for self-harm, and eliciting the details of past attempts are mandatory. The suicidal intent, i.e. the subjective expectation and desire for an attempt at self-harm to end in death, must be assessed. The lethality or the danger associated with the method used also indicates the seriousness of the person's suicidal ideation. Obtain additional information on the degree of desire to die, the intensity and frequency of suicidal ideation, ease of access to lethal methods and preparation for suicide, such as making a WILL, writing a suicide note, and making plans to avoid detection. Patients with psychotic symptoms should be asked whether they have experienced hallucinations that command them to commit suicide.

Step 2. Acknowledge distress

The elicitation of severe distress, difficult circumstances, and suicidal ideation demands empathy from the physician. Acknowledging distress is crucial in establishing a therapeutic relationship. While the availability of help should be mentioned, finding out the context, the magnitude of stress, the accessibility of resources, and the extent of support are necessary before providing reassurance, which would otherwise be premature and counterproductive. Acknowledging the distress the patient is experiencing reassures him that his cry for help has been heard. It helps to convey an empathetic attitude and establish an effective therapeutic relationship in which problems can be dealt with to facilitate improvement.

Step 3. Elicit the patient's and the family's perspective

A significant number of patients with suicidal ideation may not have a psychiatric disorder, but may be distressed by various difficulties in their lives. Asking patients what their specific concerns are allows them to talk about their distress and offers scope to suggest appropriate coping strategies. The physician should explore recent and chronic stresses in various areas, such as interpersonal problems, financial difficulties, alcohol dependence in the spouse, physical abuse, and sexual and reproductive concerns.

Step 4. Take a focused history; carry out physical examination and laboratory investigations

Patients who have attempted suicide will require a physical examination to exclude medical consequences. Those who have consumed poison and have overdosed themselves with medication will require a stomach wash, activated charcoal, and supportive measures, if they are brought within a few hours of ingestion. Monitoring their liver and kidney functions is essential.

Patients who have attempted hanging need to be evaluated for the effects of hypoxic encephalopathy; those who have swallowed corrosives require an upper gastrointestinal and a throat examination. Patients who have slashed their wrists and injured themselves will need appropriate surgical treatment and repair.

Step 5. Educate the patient and the family about attempt and ideation

Educating the patient and the family about the stress, distress, coping, and help available is crucial. Enlisting the family's support is essential. They will need to play an important role in the provision of support, monitoring of the suicidal patient, keeping him/her supervised at all times, and removing access to lethal means. If such family support is not available, the physician should consider hospitalizing the patient. Issues within the family may be the cause of conflict; in such cases, involving the family may be necessary for problem-solving.

Step 6. Prescribe medication

Patients in distress will benefit from medication. The use of vitamins as placebos is helpful in adjustment difficulties. Benzodiazepines can be employed in the short term for sleep disturbance but if the sleep problem is of long duration or if the conflicts that are causing the sleep difficulty are not going to be resolved immediately, then sedative antidepressants should be employed, as benzodiazepines are addictive.

Antidepressant medication is useful in the treatment of depression and to reduce anxiety. Newer antidepressants (e.g. selective serotonin reuptake inhibitors [SSRIs] such as fluoxetine or sertraline) are preferred when sleep is not disturbed, while small doses of tricyclic antidepressants or mirtazapine are helpful when sleep disturbance

BOX 10.1   SUICIDE ATTEMPT SECONDARY TO MELANCHOLIC DEPRESSION

A 45-year-old woman was brought to the hospital after consuming pesticide in a suicide attempt. The relatives noticed that she had been very quiet and withdrawn over the previous two months. She had a poor appetite, had lost weight, suffered from fatigue and insomnia, and had reported feeling sad, worthless, and hopeless about her life. The patient and her family did not report any psychosocial problems that had occurred in the recent times.

The patient was treated for poisoning and was started on antidepressant medication. The dose was adjusted and she was referred for counseling.

BOX 10.2   SUICIDE ATTEMPT SECONDARY TO ADJUSTMENT DIFFICULTIES

A 22-year-old man was brought to the hospital after taking an overdose of benzodiazepines following an argument with his girlfriend. He had been well until then, but just after the argument became angry and impulsively ingested the tablets that his father had kept on the bedside table.

The patient was treated for the benzodiazepine overdose. He was given time to talk about his difficulties and concerns about his relationship. He was given suggestions about ways to control his anger and impulsivity, and cope better in stressful situations. He was referred for counseling. Over time, his mental health and his relationship improved.

is present. Antipsychotics will help to reduce psychotic symptoms, while people with substance use disorders need to undergo detoxification and de-addiction. The psychiatric status and response to treatment need to be closely monitored. All medication has to be supervised, as the chances of overdose are possible.

Step 7. Discuss the role of stress as cause and consequence of problems

The role of stress, the efforts at coping with it, and its link with suicidal ideation need to be highlighted. Similarly, the consequences of the attempt in terms of immediate consequences, residual effect, hospitalization, cost, etc. should be mentioned. The fact that major damage and problems were narrowly and fortunately averted for the patient needs to be highlighted; the lack of guarantees of similar good fortune in future attempts has to be emphasized.

Step 8. Discuss coping strategies

Suggest general stress-reduction strategies. Measures such as yoga or meditation, regular physical exercise, involvement in religious activities, hobbies, and leisure all help to improve a person's coping, and are useful for those under stress.

There is a need to explore possible specific measures to reduce stress. Patients with clearly identified problems resulting in distress and suicidal ideation will need help with problem-solving. Some problems may have obvious and practical solutions. Encouraging the patient to look for specific solutions to his/her difficulties and giving him/her time to examine the issues is necessary. Other adverse life situations may be difficult to resolve and may require acceptance and a change in philosophy, attitude, and lifestyle to assist in coping. The physician's offer of psychological support is

---

**BOX 10.3   SUICIDE ATTEMPT FOLLOWING COMMAND
HALLUCINATIONS**

A 30-year-old man was brought to hospital by his family. He was diagnosed and was being treated for a chronic psychosis with antipsychotic medication. Although he had shown a reduction in his symptoms, he had discontinued treatment due to severe adverse effects. He had developed marked akathisia on 6 mg of risperidone. He had discontinued his medication and was lost to follow up. His relatives had noticed that he had become increasingly withdrawn, socially isolated, and had started talking and gesticulating to himself. He was found hanging from the ceiling in his bedroom by chance.

He was treated and management in the emergency department. His condition had stabilized and there were no major neurological deficits. He did admit to hearing voices, which commanded him to commit suicide. He said that these voices were persistent and distressing. He said that he felt powerless as the voices controlled his life. He was started on antipsychotic medication, hospitalized, and referred for psychiatric care.

necessary, while he should also encourage the patient to assume responsibility for improvement. There is a need to convey a sense of hope. Sources of strength, self-esteem, and deterrents to self-harm, such as children in the home, family relationships, religion, work, and positive support systems, need to be identified and focused upon to convey a sense of purpose. This also helps the patient focus on the positive aspects of his/her life rather than solely on the difficulties.

Step 9. Negotiate a treatment plan; discuss responsibility, participation, and compliance

In patients who are not intoxicated or psychotic, it is sometimes possible to enter into a

---

BOX 10.4   DIFFERENCE IN SUICIDE RATES

Major differences in rates of suicide and deliberate self-harm have been reported across countries, regions, cultures, and religions. While older people are at higher risk for suicide, more recently many young people seem to take their own lives. While males have a much higher rate of completed suicide, more recently the number of young women, who kill themselves, particularly in low- and middle-income countries, is increasing. Those with alcohol and substance abuse are at much greater risk for suicide and for accidental death.

People with a history of chronic pain and physical illness and those with access to medication seem to be at higher risk for suicide. Living alone, single marital status, separation, divorce, widow(er), unemployment, and homelessness also increase risk. Those with a family history of suicide have a significantly higher risk than those without. Recent bereavement also increases risk. People with a history of suicide attempts are at higher risk.

Severe mental illness has been reported in the majority of people who die by suicide in high-income countries. However, recent work from India and China has demonstrated suicide secondary to mental distress rather than among those with severe mental disorders. Countries with a good social security net and an established welfare seem to have lower rates of suicide compared to those without. People living in countries, whose economies are in transition, have a much higher risk.

Regions where firearms (e.g. USA) and lethal pesticides (e.g. farming communities in low- and middle-income countries) are easily and freely available are associated with higher rates than those without.

Suicide is the result of a complex process. There is no single cause or a specific constellation of causes, which definitely predict such death. However, a combination of high-risk factors associated with severe mental illness or distress with a lack of psychological, social, and environmental supports demand urgent intervention and care.

BOX 10.5   DIFFICULTIES IN ASSESSING SUICIDAL RISK AND CLINICAL APPROACHES TO PREVENTION

The problems in assessing suicidal risk in individuals and accurately predicting suicide are many. The very low base rate (e.g. 10 per 100,000 people) makes it difficult to study the phenomenon. Unintentional and accidental deaths are often difficult to separate from suicide and complicate its study. While many people attempt suicide and deliberate self-harm, only a minority succeed. These two groups are actually slightly overlapping populations. This makes attempting to predict suicidal risk by employing the characteristics of the dead among those living, complex and prone to error. Changes in suicidal ideation and intent over time make prediction problematic.

Many different combinations of risk factors are associated with high suicidal risk, the problems in accurate assessments, and the finality of death leaves very little room for error. Clinical approaches to assessment should aim to be highly sensitive in identifying people with high risk even if they are not specific. Consequently, it is ethically justified to intervene in the lives of many people at risk in order to prevent a few deaths.

BOX 10.6   SUPPORT FOR PHYSICIANS WHO LOST PATIENTS TO SUICIDE

Physician, psychiatrists, and mental health professionals, who care for people with chronic and severe mental disorders, are at risk for distress, when their patients commit suicide. Although such events are rare, their impact on personal and professional caregivers is significant.

Sudden loss and unexpected loss take their toll. The immediate steps would include informing your seniors at work, completing the medical records, preparing to work with the coroner or medical examiner, and contacting a trusted colleague or mentor for support.

Contacting the patient's family, emphasizing that all realistic efforts were taken to help, supporting the family through their grief, and attending the funeral, if possible, are necessary.

Discussing the issues with the mental health team, allowing for ventilation and support, doing a psychological autopsy to examine the circumstances, symptoms, and treatment procedures instituted is useful. Preparing for an audit and attempting to learn from the experience are cardinal for long-term improvement of mental healthcare for those at risk for suicide. Avoiding blaming individuals and examining the system issues is crucial for improving care.

"no-harm contract". This is an agreement between the patient and the physician wherein the patient agrees not to harm himself or herself for a specific time (e.g. 24–48 hours) and gives an assurance that he/she will contact the physician if the situation changes. This is followed up by frequent visits to the doctor or contact by telephone. The contract is renewed once the specific time period ends. Such a contract is not legally binding but may help in tiding over the acute period of crisis.

The offer of support and help also implies the need for compliance with the plan on the patient's part. The need for the patient's participation in his own recovery and the taking up of such responsibility should also be mentioned.

Step 10. Give a specific appointment for review

Regular review of progress is necessary for such patients, and appointments should be scheduled frequently during the period of acute crisis. The risk of suicide and safety issues will need to be reassessed at various points throughout treatment, as a patient's risk level will wax and wane. Some patients may be at increased risk for suicide as their energy level improves, though feelings of hopelessness and the depressed mood persist. The patient should be closely followed up and at each visit his/her progress and coping strategies should be discussed.

BOX 10.7   PUBLIC HEALTH STRATEGIES TO REDUCE SUICIDE RATES

While suicide is an individual act and requires individual assessment and management of the person, there is a need for public health measures to reduce the overall rate of suicide in populations. These measures include:

- Increasing public awareness
- Campaigning to reduce stigma associated with suicide
- Regulating formulations, packaging and sale of pesticides, and control of firearms
- Regulating sale of over-the-counter medication
- Gender-related legislation and action to prevent discrimination in patriarchal societies
- Legal issues related to suicide attempts including decriminalizing suicide attempts
- Establishing sentinel centers and developing an information system
- Training of personnel working in high-risk settings (e.g. prisons, hospitals, schools)
- Establishing crisis intervention and counseling centers and telephone hotlines
- Increasing specific clinical training programs for lay counselors
- Redesigning the curriculum for medical and nursing personnel
- Organizing intervention programs for high schools

WILL I BE ABLE TO PREVENT ALL SUICIDE ATTEMPTS?

Despite our best efforts at suicide assessment and treatment, suicides can and do occur in clinical practice. It is a relatively rare event and, therefore, difficult to accurately predict. No risk factor can be used exclusively to accurately predict suicidality. Predicting the short-term risk of a suicide attempt (in the 24- to 48-hour period after evaluation) is more reliable than predicting the long-term risk. An ongoing process of assessment is, therefore, required to prevent suicides. It is also essential to appreciate that the physician cannot solve the patient's social difficulties but can help empower patients to resolve these themselves.

WHEN SHOULD I REFER A PATIENT FOR SPECIALIST HELP?

Patients who have made a serious and lethal attempt, those with serious intent to harm themselves, and those with active plans may need to be hospitalized. People with significant distress related to stressors and those with symptoms suggestive of a severe psychiatric disorder should be referred for further treatment and hospitalization. Intoxicated or psychotic patients who say they are suicidal should also be closely supervised. The patient should not be left alone at any time, until the clinical situation has changed. Patients and families should be referred for psychological therapy to a specialist if the personality factors or stressors are severe.

Each patient will require a detailed assessment of suicidal risk. Such evaluation should allow for a stratification of risk into low, medium, and high based on their combination of risk factors, circumstances, supports, and current mental state. People with moderate to high risk will require medication and hospitalization. Those with low risk will need to have family members/carers monitor, supervise, and support them. People with moderate risk will need medication, emergency contact, and frequent and periodic reviews.

CONCLUSION

Many people experience suicidal ideation. Some of them go on to complete suicide. Therefore, suicidal ideation warrants a thorough evaluation at the time when suicidality is expressed as well as periodically thereafter. Patients who express such thoughts must be asked specific questions about recent stressors and must be evaluated for the presence of psychiatric disorders. Families should be integrated into treatment planning, which includes support, problem-solving, medication, and hospitalization, if necessary.

11 Male Sexual Dysfunction

Patients with sexual misconceptions and dysfunction frequently present to general medical settings. However, they report multiple somatic symptoms as their chief complaints. Nevertheless, they readily admit to sexual concerns on enquiry. Commonly reported problems are premature ejaculation and erectile dysfunction. The exclusion of medical causes is mandatory.

The management includes education regarding misconceptions, anatomy, and physiology of sex, contraception, and pregnancy. The need to reduce anxiety during sexual intercourse is mandatory for success. The stop–start and squeeze techniques are very useful for managing premature ejaculation, while medication such as sildenafil may be required for improving erectile function.

INTRODUCTION

Sexual dysfunctions are a heterogeneous group of disorders that produce significant disturbance in the person's ability to experience sexual pleasure or to respond sexually. Sexual response has biological underpinning but is also experienced in the intrapersonal, interpersonal, and cultural context. Therefore, sexual dysfunctions involve complex interactions among biological, psychological, and sociocultural factors.

Individuals can have one or more conditions, each of which needs to be identified and managed. While the exact etiology of various sexual dysfunctions is not known, a diagnosis of these conditions requires the exclusion of medical and neurological morbidity, or substance use. There is also a need to rule out other mental disorders.

Primary care is usually the first point of contact with health services for most people with sexual health concerns and therefore plays an important role in sexual healthcare. However, the rate of recognition and, consequently, the management, is poor. The most frequently cited reasons for this are the limitations of time and resources in primary care. Other problems include inadequate training of physicians in the recognition and management of these disorders; this, in turn, results in reduced physician confidence in dealing with such problems and reticence about discussing these issues during consultation. This chapter discusses the diagnosis and management of male sexual dysfunction in primary care and in general medical settings.

HOW DO PATIENTS WHO ATTEND PRIMARY CARE MANIFEST THEIR SEXUAL PROBLEMS?

Patients rarely report sexual dysfunction as the reason for consultation. The majority of patients with such problems present with physical symptoms such as weakness, fatigue, aches and pains, or other medically unexplained physical symptoms. A small proportion of subjects may present with depression, marital discord, or substance abuse. It is rare for men to directly present with complaints of sexual dysfunction.

WHAT ARE THE COMMON SEXUAL DISORDERS SEEN IN PRIMARY CARE?

Erectile dysfunction and premature ejaculation are the common male sexual disorders encountered in primary care. Orgasmic dysfunction (delayed or retarded ejaculation, anejaculation, or anorgasmia), low sexual desire, and sexual aversion are less frequently reported. Issues with regard to sexual orientation and sexual preference are not commonly seen in primary care unless these are in combination with common psychiatric presentations.

HOW COMMON ARE SEXUAL DISORDERS IN PRIMARY CARE?

Studies from the West and some Asian countries report the prevalence as ranging from 30%–60% in men. There is a significant age-related correlation in the prevalence of sexual dysfunctions, particularly after the age of 50 years.

IF PEOPLE WITH SEXUAL DISORDERS PRESENT TO PRIMARY CARE, WHY IS IT DIFFICULT TO RECOGNIZE AND MANAGE THESE IN CLINICAL PRACTICE?

There are many reasons as to why sexual problems are under-recognized in primary care. These include the reluctance of patients and physicians to discuss sexual issues, which are considered sensitive or embarrassing, the perception that sexual problems are not "serious", and inadequate physician skill and confidence in managing these problems. Excessive reliance on culturally acceptable, traditional forms of treatments offered by traditional healers and alternative systems of medicine often leads to under-reporting of these symptoms in medical settings.

WHAT QUESTIONS CAN I ASK THE PATIENT TO ELICIT SEXUAL PROBLEMS?

The first step in assessing sexual dysfunction is to establish rapport and ensure non-judgmental, respectful communication regarding sexuality. The language must be simple and appropriate to the local culture. Open-ended questions, such as "Do you have any sexual concerns?", "Are you satisfied with your current sexual functioning?", or "How is your sex life?" will encourage the patient to talk about these problems. Direct questions can put patients at ease by indicating that the doctor is willing to discuss issues related to sex. While there may be initial inhibition, most patients are willing to discuss their sexual problems and, in fact, may be waiting to mention them to the physician, if given an opportunity. Providing privacy encourages disclosure. Specific questions to elicit erectile dysfunction and premature ejaculation such as "Do you have trouble getting or keeping an erection?", and "Do you or your partner feel that you ejaculate too quickly?" are useful.

HOW DO I MAKE A DIAGNOSIS?

Premature ejaculation is considered when the patient reports ejaculation that occurs sooner than desired, either before or shortly after penetration, causing distress to either one or both partners. Literature is replete with attempts to ascertain a time limit to make a diagnosis of premature ejaculation. However, clinically the most important criteria for a diagnosis would be the patient's and/or partner's distress.

Erectile dysfunction is the inability to achieve or maintain an erection sufficient for intercourse when attempted. It is useful to differentiate between a disorder that has been lifelong and one of recent onset, as well as between dysfunction that occurs globally and that which occurs in specific situations or with specific partners.

WHAT ARE THE COMMON CAUSES OF SEXUAL DYSFUNCTION?

Sexual dysfunction is best described as multifactorial in origin with organic and psychogenic causes, though, in some cases, it may be a combination. Table 11.1 provides a simple guide to distinguish between these two groups.

While a multifactorial etiology in the causation of erectile dysfunction with both medical and psychological causes contributing is common, the differentiation can be clinically helpful. Psychological causation demands the transfer of skill and confidence to the patient, while medical causation mandates treatment of the cause and medication.

CAN MEDICAL CAUSES BE IDENTIFIED BY HISTORY AND CLINICAL EXAMINATION?

A detailed history and clinical examination are useful in ruling out common medical causes of sexual dysfunction. Physical factors that contribute to sexual dysfunction are listed in Table 11.2.

TABLE 11.1

Some Pointers that Help Distinguish between Organic and Psychogenic Causes of Erectile Dysfunction

Characteristic	Organic cause	Psychogenic problem
Age	Older	Younger
Age of onset of problem	Late-age onset	Onset in adolescence/ adulthood
Onset	Often insidious	Usually acute
Specificity of dysfunction	Usually global	Usually partner- or situation-specific
Premature ejaculation	Usually absent	Often present
Nocturnal penile tumescence	Usually absent	Usually present
Medical illness and medication for disease	Usually present	Usually absent
Neurological deficits, bowel and bladder problems	May be present	Usually absent
Performance and spectator anxiety	Usually absent	Usually present
History of surgery or trauma (abdominal or spinal)	May be present	Usually absent

---

TABLE 11.2

Common Physical Disorders that can Manifest with Sexual Disorders

1. *Vascular Disorders:* hypertension, diabetes mellitus, dyslipidaemias, cardiovascular disease
2. *Neurogenic Damage:* cerebrovascular accidents, peripheral neuropathy, spinal cord damage
3. *Hormonal Problems:* hypogonadism, hyper/hypothyroidism, hyperglycemia
4. *Iatrogenic Causes:* post-radiation, postoperative, medication-induced (antihypertensives, psychotropics, diuretics, opioids, etc.)

HOW SHOULD I PROCEED?

Once sexual dysfunction is established, comorbid medical illnesses (Table 11.2) must be evaluated for, along with a focused physical examination and relevant investigations. Details of medication that the patient is currently on must be elicited as these may sometimes contribute to sexual dysfunction. The history of psychiatric disorders and other psychological and social difficulties in the patient's life must be explored. Misconceptions and doubts about sex and sexual function should be elicited and clarified (Table 11.3).

TABLE 11.3

Common Misconceptions, Situations, and Anxieties Causing Sexual Dysfunction

Personal Situations
- after prolonged periods of abstinence
- physical exhaustion
- use of alcohol
- during periods of stress and worry
- discord with partner (e.g. marital discord)

Circumstances of Sexual Intercourse
- lack of privacy
- lack of contraception and the fear of pregnancy
- failure to use a condom and fear of getting/transferring sexually transmitted disease
- context of an "illicit" relationship and fear of getting "caught"
- putting oneself to the "test" after a history of dysfunction

Issues Directly Related to Sexual Intercourse
- inadequate foreplay leading to poor lubrication and painful intercourse
- refractory phase of the sexual cycle
- spectator anxiety focusing on oneself from a third-person perspective during sexual activity, rather than focusing on one's sensations and/or sexual partner

Misconceptions or Lack of Knowledge
- related to structure (shape, size) and function of genitalia (e.g. fears related to "loss of semen", nocturnal emission, masturbatory guilt)
- poor understanding of the nature/unrealistic expectation of sexual intercourse
- misconceptions related to pregnancy, contraception, etc.

People with sexual dysfunction often have problems in several spheres of life. These include marital and relationship difficulties, low self-esteem, and substance use disorders. These patients may also develop common mental disorders, such as depression, anxiety, and medically unexplained symptoms, which can cause significant socio-occupational dysfunction. A large number may seek traditional healing and alternative therapies to overcome their difficulties.

WHAT IS THE BASIS OF THE SUGGESTED PROTOCOL?

This protocol is adapted from the PLISSIT (**P**ermission, **L**imited **I**nformation, **S**pecific **S**uggestions, **I**ntensive **T**herapy) model, which is a behavioral approach for managing sexual dysfunction. It has been modified to incorporate the cultural needs of different populations and recent advances in this field. The steps, the sequence, and their rationale are briefly described.

WHAT ARE THE STEPS IN THE PROTOCOL?

The ten steps in management are:

1. Recognize the clinical presentation
2. Acknowledge distress
3. Elicit the patient's and the family's perspective
4. Take a focused history; carry out physical examination and laboratory investigations
5. Educate the patient about the nature of illness and its treatment
6. Prescribe medication
7. Discuss the role of stress as cause and consequence of illness
8. Elaborate coping strategies
9. Negotiate a treatment plan, compliance, participation, and responsibility
10. Give a specific appointment for review.

Step 1. Recognize the clinical presentation

Very few patients directly present with complaints of sexual dysfunction because of the cultural inhibitions regarding talking about sex; the vast majority present with medically unexplained somatic complaints, alcohol abuse, or marital discord. However, eliciting underlying sexual problems is easy with direct questions. Recognizing the common clinical presentations of premature ejaculation and erectile dysfunction is crucial.

Step 2. Acknowledge distress

Patients may be distressed because of the incapacitating nature of their sexual problems, their inability to discuss the issue with peers because of embarrassment and the impact on their relationships. Acknowledging the distress caused by the sexual problems reassures the patient and helps establish rapport, which is essential for a therapeutic relationship and in facilitating improvement. The failure to do so, along with premature reassurance, reinforces the patient's belief that the physician does not understand the seriousness of the problem.

Step 3. Elicit the patient's and the family's perspective

Providing appropriate reassurance is an important part of medical consultation. It is most effective if based on the patient's actual concerns. Asking patients what they think or fear is the cause of the dysfunction is useful in addressing specific concerns (e.g. "It is because of excessive loss of semen due to masturbation"). Many beliefs and misconceptions held by patients may increase stress and consequently undermine sexual performance. The belief that "loss of semen" (e.g. dhat syndrome in the south Asian culture) is the cause of symptoms such as weakness, fatigue, and memory loss are common. Practitioners of traditional systems of medicine and healing, who subscribe to these concepts and who are often the first contacts in the "pathway to care", often reinforce such beliefs.

The patient's beliefs need to be discussed before presenting alternative biomedical explanation. An outright rejection of the patient's beliefs about his illness early in the consultation or a failure to elicit them often proves disastrous. Eliciting such explanations will also allow for focused examination, investigations, and specific reassurance.

Step 4. Take a focused history; carry out physical examination and laboratory investigations

Satisfaction with current sexual functioning needs to be enquired into. If there is a problem, the duration and nature of the dysfunction must be identified. Common areas of dysfunction include little or no interest in sex, problems in achieving erection, ejaculating too early during sexual activity, taking too long to ejaculate, inability to ejaculate or have an orgasm, pain during sex, and penile curvature during erection.

Attempting to understand the patient's social and cultural background, relationships, perceptions about normal sexuality, sexual orientation and preferences, psychosocial stressors, and sexual misconceptions is important in understanding and managing sexual dysfunction. Common mental disorders such as anxiety, depression, and substance use disorders, which contribute to sexual dysfunction, must be identified and managed. It is useful to understand how the client's sexual difficulties started and past treatments that he has had, in order to formulate a plan.

A focused physical examination (including genital examination) is cardinal for identifying sexual disorders that are secondary to physical disease or substance abuse. Physical factors, which contribute to sexual dysfunction, are listed in Table 11.2. A good physical examination is also essential to help clarify misconceptions that the patient may have regarding the sexual organs. Basic laboratory investigations should be ordered (e.g. blood sugar, serum lipid profile, complete blood count, serum creatinine, etc.) while special tests (e.g. serum prolactin, testosterone, androgens) may be required for those with endocrine problems. An electrocardiogram is mandatory in the older age group, especially when using phosphodiesterase inhibitors. Managing medical causes optimally is obligatory.

Step 5. Educate the patient about the nature of illness and treatment

Many individuals experience sexual problems secondary to sexual misconceptions, unrealistic expectations, doubts, and fears (Table 11.3). Clarifications about normal sexual function, pregnancy, contraception, and sexually transmitted infections often relieve distress and improve sexual performance. Simple advice can make a huge difference to the outcome. Avoiding personal situations where dysfunction is common is useful (e.g. in situations where there is no privacy). Giving reassurance about normal structure and function and discussing the issues related to the circumstances go a long way in clarifying misconceptions, reducing fears and anxieties, and increasing performance. Advice on contraception to prevent pregnancy and the use of condoms to prevent sexually transmitted infections helps people with these concerns. Avoiding sexual intercourse in situations where there is a fear of detection reduces the chances of dysfunction. Advice on reducing or eliminating these difficulties is often an adequate solution for many people with sexual dysfunction. This step is useful in the manipulation of personal and environmental factors, which can have a major impact on the patient's sexual functioning.

The problem of premature ejaculation can be easily addressed in primary care. The "squeeze technique" (i.e. application of gentle pressure on the glans penis by compression between thumb and fingers before the threshold of ejaculatory inevitability is reached) can be taught. This helps to delay ejaculation and prolong sexual intercourse. This is also called the "start–stop technique" as the male needs to interrupt intercourse to delay ejaculation.

Step 6. Prescribe medication

Many patients benefit with just a clarification of their misconceptions. Premature ejaculation requires the use of the simple techniques mentioned above and usually does not require medication.

Small doses of antidepressants such as clomipramine (25–50 mg), imipramine (20–50 mg), or sertraline (25–50 mg) are helpful in managing the symptoms of anxiety and depression seen in many people with sexual dysfunction. These also have a beneficial effect in patients with premature ejaculation as these drugs also delay ejaculation; however, at higher doses they may worsen erectile dysfunction.

Phosphodiestrase inhibitors, such as sildenafil and tadalafil, have been shown to be effective in the management of erectile dysfunction of varying etiology. Table 11.4 compares these medications. These drugs have also been shown to be beneficial in premature ejaculation and improving sexual desire disorders in men.

Step 7. Discuss the role of stress as a cause or consequence

Stress in the environment, at work, and at home can result in sexual dysfunction. Misconceptions are also a major cause of psychological stress and place unrealistic demands, leading to increased psychological tension. Sexual dysfunction itself increases anxiety and distress in individuals, setting up a vicious cycle and perpetuating sexual problems.

TABLE 11.4

Phosphodiestrase Inhibitors Commonly Used in the Treatment of Erectile Dysfunction

Characteristics	Sildenafil	Tadalafil
Onset of action	Less than 40 minutes	Less than 40 minutes
Duration of action	Up to 4 hours	36 hours or more
Administration – with food – with high-fat meals	Can be administered Slows absorption	Can be administered No effect on absorption
Usual dose	25–100 mg	5–20 mg
Dose in special circumstances – renal impairment – hepatic impairment – elderly	Low doses Low doses Low doses	Low doses Low doses* Normal dose
Concomitant medications – nitrates – strong CYP3A4 inhibitors – class Ia and III anti-arrhythmic agents	Contraindicated Reduce dose Can be used	Contraindicated Reduce dose Can be used
Common side-effects	Headache Flushing Dyspepsia Nasal congestion Altered vision	Headache Flushing Dyspepsia Nasal congestion Visual disturbances Myalgia and back pain

* Not recommended in severe hepatic impairment

BOX 11.1   ANXIETY AND PREMATURE EJACULATION

A 30-year-old married man presented with a history of abdominal pain. He had been evaluated in many hospitals and all his investigations were normal. On enquiry, he mentioned that he had problems during sexual intercourse and that he would ejaculate prematurely, before he and his wife could achieve orgasm and satisfaction.

He was educated about the nature of his problem. Anatomy, physiology, contraception, and issues related to pregnancy were discussed. Sexual misconceptions were elicited and corrected. He was advised to avoid watching his performance during sex. He was taught the stop–start and squeeze techniques. He was also started on a small dose of tab. imipramine 25 mg, at bedtime. He gained confidence, recovered his function, and the medication was stopped in two months.

Step 8. Elaborate coping strategies

Sexual dysfunction may be secondary to marital discord, anxiety, or poor sexual technique. Specific suggestions help individuals reach goals such as improved communication, reduction in anxiety, or the learning of new arousal behaviors. Discussing the need to improve the marital relationship and bring back the romance can help couples with marital discord. Yoga and meditation are general measures that are helpful in reducing anxiety. Men mostly become extremely anxious due to the "pressure to perform" following previous failures during sexual intercourse that could have been due to a variety of reasons. Measures to specifically reduce anxiety during sexual intercourse include increasing the duration of foreplay, reducing the focus on genital contact, preventing "spectator anxiety", and focusing on pleasure rather than performance.

Step 9. Negotiate a treatment plan, compliance, participation, and responsibility

While the physician can help in excluding medical causes of sexual dysfunction, clarifying sexual misconceptions, suggesting simple techniques to improve function, and prescribing medication, the patient will have to implement the many suggestions for success. Consequently, there is a need to negotiate a plan of action, and discuss patient participation, responsibility, and compliance with medication, and psychological and sexual advice.

Step 10. Give a specific appointment for review

Regular review of progress is necessary for most patients and there should be scheduled, brief appointments every 2–4 weeks (i.e. avoiding "as-needed" appointments). These sessions should be utilized to assess the progress made and identify new difficulties. The physician's approach at these sessions should be of a "cheer-leader" who provides encouragement and specific suggestions.

BOX 11.2   ERECTILE DYSFUNCTION

A 40-year-old married man was diagnosed to have diabetes and was on oral hypoglycemic medication. On enquiry, he mentioned that he had problems during sexual intercourse and that he would achieve inadequate erection for successful sexual intercourse. His blood sugars were under control and he did not have peripheral or autonomic neuropathy.

He was educated about the nature of his problem. Anatomy, physiology, contraception, and issues related to pregnancy were discussed. He was started on tab. sildenafil 25 mg, and was advised to take it an hour before intercourse. This resulted in an improved but less than normal performance. The dose of sildenafil was increased to 50 mg. He gained confidence, recovered his function, and the medication was gradually tapered and stopped in two months.

BOX 11.3   OTHER FACTORS IN ETIOLOGY OF SEXUAL DYSFUNCTION

A number of other factors can be associated with a person's sexual dysfunction. These may be relevant to the etiology and may contribute to varying degrees. They may also be crucial in management. Some are listed below:

- *Partner Factors*
  - Partner's sexual problems
  - Partner's health status
- *Relationship Factors*
  - Poor communication
  - Discrepancies in desire for sexual activity
- *Individual Vulnerability Issues*
  - Poor body image
  - History of sexual abuse
  - History of emotional abuse
  - Psychiatric comorbidity (e.g. anxiety, depression)
  - Stressors (e.g. loss of employment, bereavement)
- *Cultural or Religious Factors*
  - Attitudes towards sexuality
  - Inhibitions to religious or cultural prohibitions against sexual activity/ pleasure
- *Medical Concerns*
  - Medical comorbidity
  - Medication induced sexual dysfunction

BOX 11.4   THE MAGNITUDE OF SEXUAL PROBLEMS

Prior to the success of Viagra (sildenafil citrate), sexual dysfunction remained hidden. Massive profits for Pfizer, its manufacturers, suggested that they had identified a significant felt need. The publicity surrounding the drug resulted in a public debate about erectile dysfunction, sex, and sexuality.

The high prevalence of sexual misconceptions and dysfunction in the general population demands that physicians and counselors explore sex and sexuality and recognize disorders and disability with a view to address them.

WILL I BE ABLE TO DO THIS IN MY BUSY CLINICAL PRACTICE?

Physicians often worry that managing sexual problems requires specific skill and takes time. The majority of people with sexual dysfunction require clarification of misconceptions, education on normal sexual function, and simple advice on avoiding circumstances that cause difficulties. The squeeze technique is easily taught using simple diagrams and is effective in reducing premature ejaculation and in increasing performance over time. The newer drugs are very effective in a variety of dysfunctions of organic, psychological, and mixed etiologies.

The primary job of a physician is to clarify issues, provide targeted solutions, and instill confidence in the patient. With practice, the efficiency of the technique used improves and such counseling can be used in real-life situations in a session of 10–15 minutes.

WHEN SHOULD I REFER A PATIENT FOR SPECIALIST HELP?

Sexual orientation/preference issues, severe marital discord, comorbid substance use, or major psychiatric disorders may necessitate a psychiatric consultation. Uncontrolled diabetes or hypertension, medication-induced sexual dysfunction, or structural organic conditions may also need specialist intervention. It is useful to refer patients who have not benefited from treatment in primary care for specialist intervention.

CONCLUSION

Sexual dysfunction is a common problem; however, it is rarely discussed or managed in primary care. It is essential that the physician is comfortable discussing these issues with patients to allow for appropriate intervention and management.

12 Female Sexual Dysfunction

Women who present with multiple somatic complaints can have sexual concerns and dysfunction as the stressors causing their symptoms. Lack of interest in or desire for sex is the most common sexual problem among women. Other common problems include difficulty becoming or remaining aroused during sexual activity, difficulty in achieving orgasm, pain associated with sexual stimulation, concerns about vaginal discharge, and fear of pregnancy and delivery. These concerns may be associated with marital discord.

The management includes the elicitation of problems, understanding the context, education about misconceptions and sexual function, and advice on contraception and pregnancy. Marital and other conflicts will require resolution. Medication may also be required for the treatment of anxiety and depressive symptoms.

INTRODUCTION

Sexual dysfunction in women is a group of heterogeneous conditions. However, cultural factors often result in their under-reporting, under-diagnosis, and the consequent failure to recognize their impact on the lives of women.

Primary care is usually the first point of contact with health services for most people with sexual health concerns. However, the rate of recognition, and consequently the management, is even more dismal for women with sexual problems than for men. This is consequent to inadequate training of physicians in the recognition and management of these disorders and reticence in discussing these issues during consultation, which is more so in the case of women. There is great variability in sexual interest and response among women. A dysfunction is assumed when the woman is unable to participate in a sexual relationship, as she would wish. This chapter discusses the diagnosis and management of female sexual dysfunction in primary care and in general medical settings.

HOW DO WOMEN WHO ATTEND PRIMARY CARE MANIFEST THEIR SEXUAL PROBLEMS?

Patients rarely report sexual dysfunction as the reason for consultation. The majority of patients with such problems present with physical symptoms, such as weakness, fatigue, aches and pains, or other medically unexplained physical symptoms. A small proportion of subjects may present with depression, marital discord, or substance abuse.

WHAT ARE THE COMMON FEMALE SEXUAL DISORDERS SEEN IN PRIMARY CARE?

Lack of interest in or desire for sex is the most common sexual problem among women. Other common problems include difficulty becoming or remaining aroused during sexual activity, difficulty in achieving orgasm, pain associated with sexual stimulation, concerns about vaginal discharge, and fear of pregnancy and delivery. Several of these problems may also occur together. Issues with regard to sexual orientation and sexual preference are less commonly seen in primary care.

HOW COMMON ARE FEMALE SEXUAL DISORDERS IN PRIMARY CARE?

Studies from the West and Asian countries report the prevalence of female sexual dysfunction as ranging from 43% to 63%.

IF WOMEN WITH SEXUAL DISORDERS PRESENT TO PRIMARY CARE, WHY IS IT DIFFICULT TO RECOGNIZE AND MANAGE THESE IN CLINICAL PRACTICE?

There are many reasons as to why sexual problems are under-recognized in primary care. These include the reluctance of patients and physicians to discuss sexual issues, which are considered sensitive or embarrassing, the perception that sexual problems are not "serious", or that it is inappropriate or shameful for women to be concerned about sexual matters, as well as inadequate physician skill and confidence in managing these problems. Excessive reliance on culturally acceptable, traditional forms of treatment such as those offered by traditional healers and alternative systems of medicine, often leads to under-reporting of these symptoms in medical settings.

WHAT QUESTIONS CAN I ASK THE PATIENT TO ELICIT SEXUAL PROBLEMS?

The first step in assessing sexual dysfunction is to establish rapport and ensure non-judgmental, respectful communication regarding sexuality. The language used must be simple and appropriate for the local culture. Open-ended questions, such as "Do you have any sexual concerns?", "Are you satisfied with your current sexual functioning?", or "How is your sex life?" will encourage the patient to talk about these problems. Direct questions can put patients at ease by indicating that the doctor is willing to discuss issues related to sex. While there may be initial inhibition, most patients are willing to discuss their sexual problems and, in fact, may be waiting to mention them to the physician if given an opportunity. Providing privacy encourages disclosure.

HOW DO I MAKE A DIAGNOSIS?

Sexual desire disorders are a common problem, where the individual has a lack or loss of sexual desire and is not interested in initiating sexual activity. Patients may also report an aversion to and avoidance of genital contact with the partner; this is termed as sexual aversion disorder. In disorders of sexual arousal, the desire for sex might be intact, but the individual has difficulty attaining or maintaining vaginal lubrication during sexual activity. Anorgasmia is described as a difficulty in achieving orgasm despite sufficient sexual interest, stimulation, and arousal.

What are the common causes of female sexual dysfunction?

Female sexual dysfunction is best described as multifactorial in origin, with organic and psychogenic causes, though in some cases it may be a combination.

Can medical causes be identified by history and clinical examination?

A detailed history and clinical examination are useful in ruling out common medical and gynecological causes of sexual dysfunction. The physical factors that contribute to sexual dysfunction are listed in Table 12.1.

How should I proceed?

Once sexual dysfunction is established by obtaining a detailed patient history, comorbid medical or gynecological illnesses (Table 12.1) must be evaluated for, along with a focused physical and gynecological examination and relevant investigations. Details of medication that the patient is currently on must be elicited as these may sometimes contribute to sexual dysfunction. The possibility of psychiatric disorders and other psychological and social difficulties in the patient's life must be explored. Misconceptions and doubts about sex and sexual function should be elicited and clarified (Table 12.2).

What happens to patients who do not get help from physicians?

Women with sexual dysfunction often have problems in other spheres of life, most commonly marital and relationship difficulties. They may also develop common mental disorders, such as depression, anxiety, and medically unexplained symptoms, which can cause significant socio-occupational dysfunction. Some may seek alternative therapies to overcome their difficulties.

What is the basis of the suggested protocol?

This protocol is adapted from the PLISSIT (**P**ermission, **L**imited **I**nformation, **S**pecific

---

TABLE 12.1

Common Physical Disorders that can Manifest with Sexual Disorders

- *Vascular Disorders:* hypertension, diabetes mellitus, dyslipidemias, cardiovascular disease
- *Neurogenic Damage:* cerebrovascular accidents, peripheral neuropathy, spinal cord damage, multiple sclerosis, Parkinson disease, head injury, epilepsy, tumors
- *Bone and Joint Problems:* arthritis
- *Hormonal Problems:* thyroid disorders, diabetes, pituitary disorders
- *Gynecological Problems:* vaginitis, pelvic inflammatory disease, endometriosis, fibroids, prolapse uterus, urinary incontinence; gynecological changes related to a woman's reproductive life (e.g. puberty, pregnancy, the postpartum period and menopause)
- *Iatrogenic Causes:* post-radiation, postoperative (oophorectomy, episiotomy, mastectomy, colostomy), medication-induced (antihypertensives, anticholinergics, psychotropics, diuretics, opioids, etc.)
- *Substance Abuse Problems:* alcohol, nicotine, benzodiazepines, opioids

---

TABLE 12.2

Common Misconceptions, Situations, and Anxieties causing Sexual Dysfunction

- *Personal Situations*
  - physical exhaustion
  - use of alcohol or other substances of abuse
  - during periods of stress and worry
  - discord with partner (e.g. marital discord)

- *Circumstances of Sexual Intercourse*
  - lack of privacy
  - lack of contraception and the fear of pregnancy
  - failure of spouse to use a condom and fear of getting/transferring sexually transmitted disease
  - context of an "illicit" relationship and fear of getting "caught"

- *Issues Directly Related to Sexual Intercourse*
  - inadequate foreplay leading to poor lubrication and painful intercourse
  - spectator anxiety with the patient focusing on herself from a third-person perspective during sexual activity, rather than focusing on her sensations and/or sexual partner

- *Misconceptions or Lack of Knowledge*
  - related to structure and function of genitalia
  - poor understanding of the nature/unrealistic expectation of sexual intercourse
  - misconceptions related to menstruation, pregnancy, contraception, etc.

Suggestions, Intensive Therapy) model, which is a behavioral approach to managing sexual dysfunction. If the physician enquires about sexual function during the clinical encounter, it validates sexuality as a legitimate health issue and gives the patient permission to discuss her sexual concerns. The model suggests a stepwise approach to addressing sexual concerns. Some problems can be sorted if the physician addresses specific sexual concerns and attempts to correct myths and misinformation by providing limited information. Other more complex dysfunctions require greater understanding of the issues and specific suggestions to address particular issues, define appropriate goals, and consider treatment plans. Finally, the protocol provides for intensive therapy or specialized treatment if permission, limited information, and specific suggestions have not helped.

While the principles of the model are well established, they will need to be tailored to meet the social and cultural context. The steps, the sequence, and their rationale are briefly described.

WHAT ARE THE STEPS IN THE PROTOCOL?

The ten steps in management are:

1. Recognize the clinical presentation
2. Acknowledge distress
3. Elicit the patient's and the family's perspective
4. Take a focused history; carry out physical examination and laboratory investigations
5. Educate the patient about the nature of illness and its treatment

6. Prescribe medication
7. Discuss the role of stress as cause and consequence of illness
8. Elaborate coping strategies
9. Negotiate a treatment plan, compliance, participation, and responsibility
10. Give an appointment for review.

Step 1. Recognize the clinical presentation

Very few women directly present with complaints of sexual dysfunction because of the inhibitions in the culture about talking about sex. The majority of women, who attend primary care, highlight somatic symptoms as their reason for the consultation. Some women might mention marital discord and emotional distress. However, eliciting underlying sexual problems is easy with direct questions. Recognizing the common clinical presentations of lack of interest in sex, difficulties in arousal and orgasm, or pain related to sexual activity is important.

Step 2. Acknowledge distress

Patients are often distressed by sexual problems, their inability to discuss the issue with peers because of embarrassment and the impact it has on their relationships. Acknowledging the distress caused by these sexual problems reassures the patient, reflects an empathetic attitude, and conveys a willingness to discuss the problem. It also helps establish a rapport, which is essential for a therapeutic relationship, and in facilitating improvement. The failure to do so, along with premature reassurance, reinforces the patient's beliefs that the physician has not understood the seriousness of the problem.

Step 3. Elicit the patient's and the family's perspective

Providing appropriate reassurance is an important part of the medical consultation. It is most effective if based on the patient's actual concerns. Asking the patient what she thinks or fears may be the cause of dysfunction is essential in addressing specific concerns and in providing appropriate reassurance (e.g. "I think my problems are due to my irregular periods"). Many individuals experience sexual problems secondary to misconceptions that may increase stress and consequently sexual performance. Such misconceptions are usually related to anatomy and physiology, lack of knowledge, and unrealistic expectations and fears related to sexuality and sexual functions. Fears related to pregnancy, lack of contraception, unprotected sex, and negative feelings (shame, guilt, fear, and anger) about sex due to cultural/religious factors or past sexual trauma are common problems among women with sexual dysfunction. Some women may experience a loss of self-esteem or a fear of discomfort following surgical procedures such as mastectomy or colostomy.

The patient's beliefs need to be discussed before presenting alternative biomedical explanations. Outright rejection of the patient's beliefs about her illness early in the consultation or a failure to elicit them often proves disastrous. Eliciting such explanations will also allow for focused examination, investigations, and specific reassurance.

Step 4. Take a focused history; carry out physical examination and laboratory investigations

Satisfaction with current sexual functioning needs to be enquired into. The sexual dysfunction should be defined in terms of nature, onset, duration, and whether the problem is situational – with a specific partner, setting, or circumstance – or global. Long-standing issues need to be differentiated from those of more recent onset.

Attempting to understand the patient's social and cultural background, the quality of her relationships, her perceptions about normal sexuality, and her sexual orientation and preferences is important for an appreciation of the possible cause of the sexual dysfunction.

Common mental disorders such as anxiety, depression, and substance use disorders, which contribute to sexual dysfunction, must be identified and managed.

A focused physical examination, including a genital and pelvic examination, is necessary to identify sexual disorders that are secondary to physical disease (Table 12.1), as well as to help clarify misconceptions that the patient may have regarding the sexual organs. Local problems that commonly result in pain and decreased arousal in women include pelvic infections, cysts or tumors, endometriosis, painful scars in the vaginal region due to injury, childbirth or surgery and irritation from local applications, spermicides, or latex in condoms. Medical conditions such as diabetes mellitus, multiple sclerosis, and Crohn disease can affect sexual desire and arousal. Medication that might contribute to loss of sexual desire and inability to achieve orgasm include antidepressants, antipsychotic medications, antihypertensives, hormonal contraceptives, and H2 blockers; excessive use of alcohol and drug abuse may also add to the problems. Basic laboratory tests should be ordered (e.g. complete blood count, blood sugar levels, lipid levels, and serum creatinine), while special tests (e.g. thyroid function tests, prolactin, follicle-stimulating hormone, luteinizing hormone levels) may be required for those with endocrine problems. It is essential to manage and treat medical causes optimally.

In the absence of medical disease, female sexual problems are most likely to be secondary to psychosocial and emotional problems, such as a poor relationship with the partner, and common mental disorders such as anxiety and depression.

Step 5. Educate the patient about the nature of illness and treatment

Many individuals experience sexual problems secondary to sexual misconceptions, unrealistic expectations, doubts, and fears (Table 12.2). Educating the patient about the normal structure and function of the genitals, normal sexual function, pregnancy, and the normal changes of aging and menopause often relieve distress and improve sexual performance. Contraception to prevent pregnancy and the use of condoms to prevent sexually transmitted infection, help people with these concerns. Avoiding personal situations where dysfunction is common, such as situations where there is a fear of detection, reduces the chances of dysfunction. Possible explanations for the patient's symptoms (such as stress, marital discord, and unrealistic expectations) are useful. For reassurance to be effective, the patient's specific concerns need to be elicited and appropriate explanations provided.

Step 6. Prescribe medication

Many patients benefit with just a clarification of their misconceptions and reassurance. Others with pain and problems with lubrication can benefit with specific suggestions. However, some patients may require small doses of antidepressants, such as dosulepin/ dothiepin (25–50 mg) or sertraline (25–50 mg), to manage symptoms of anxiety and depression. Underlying medical problems and substance use disorders that contribute to sexual dysfunction must be identified and treated appropriately. Although flibanserin has been recently approved for the treatment of female sexual dysfunction, the jury is still out on its usefulness in routine clinical practice.

Step 7. Discuss the role of stress as a cause and consequence of illness

The stress of daily living, including concerns about work, family, and finances, can result in anxiety that affects sexual functioning. Interpersonal conflicts in the marital relationship can affect sexual responsiveness. Sexual misconceptions are also a major cause of psychological stress and place unrealistic demands, leading to increased psychological tension.

Sexual dysfunction itself increases the anxiety and stress in individuals, which sets up a vicious cycle and perpetuates sexual problems. Helping the patient to understand the relationship between emotional factors and her physical concerns is an important step.

BOX 12.1 SOME DESCRIPTIONS

Lack or Loss of Sexual Desire: There is a lack or loss of sexual desire, evident by a reduction of feelings of desire on thinking about sex or sexual fantasies. There is a lack of interest in initiating sexual activity, resulting in a reduced frequency of sexual activity.

Sexual Aversion: The thought of sexual interaction produces such an aversion, fear, or anxiety that sexual activity is avoided, or is associated with strong negative feelings and an inability to experience any pleasure.

Sexual Arousal Disorder: There is a failure to experience adequate vaginal lubrication, together with inadequate tumescence of the labia during sexual activity.

Orgasmic Dysfunction: There is either absence or marked delay of orgasm (the moment of most intense pleasure in sexual intercourse) during sexual activity.

Vaginismus: There is a spasm of the perivaginal muscles, which prevents penile entry or makes it uncomfortable; therefore, any attempt at sexual contact leads to generalized fear and efforts to avoid it.

Dyspareunia: Pain is experienced in the vagina during sexual intercourse that is not due to vaginismus or failure of lubrication.

Step 8. Elaborate coping strategies

Sexual dysfunction may be secondary to marital discord, anxiety, or poor sexual technique. Specific suggestions help individuals reach goals such as improved communication, reduction in anxiety or learning of new arousal behaviors. Improving communication between the couple, reducing conflict, and bringing back the romance in the relationship can help couples with marital discord. Anxiety can inhibit sexual arousal; strategies to alleviate anxiety include employing distraction techniques, reducing the focus on genital contact, and focusing on pleasure rather than performance. General psychological measures, such as practicing yoga and meditation, and regular physical exercise or involvement in leisure, hobbies or religious activities are helpful in reducing anxiety.

Other specific measures to improve sexual functioning in women include encouraging open communication between the couple about likes and dislikes during sexual activity, increasing the duration of foreplay to increase stimulation and arousal,

---

BOX 12.2   SEXUAL MISCONCEPTIONS AND PROBLEMS

A 32-year-old housewife was brought to the doctor by her husband, with the chief complaint of infrequent sexual interaction. The couple was otherwise happy and committed to each other. On further evaluation, the husband reported episodes of premature ejaculation and said his anxiety about this made him inhibited about seeking sexual contact with his wife. The patient reported that while she cared for her husband, she felt unattractive and especially found her genitalia repulsive. She also believed that sex was dirty and it was wrong to enjoy coitus. The patient had a sexual aversion and several misconceptions about sexuality, while her husband was diagnosed to have premature ejaculation.

Both partners were allowed to express their distress and their concepts, beliefs, and expectations regarding sex. The patient reported that she had been brought up in a very conservative home where sex was considered taboo and, therefore, had a very negative view about sex and sexuality. A focused physical and genital examination as well as laboratory investigations for both partners did not reveal any abnormality. She was educated about the normal structure and function of the genitals with simple pictures and diagrams, and she was encouraged to re-evaluate her perception of her genitals as ugly. Her concerns regarding the morals of sex were discussed. She was reassured that enjoying sex with her husband was not wrong but normal and that she had society's permission to do so. The couple was educated about how the stress related to the patient's misconceptions and the husband's anxiety regarding his performance were increasing their sexual problems. The couple was encouraged to improve communication between them, reduce the focus on genital contact, increase the duration of foreplay, and focus on pleasure rather than performance. They were taught the "squeeze" technique to deal with the husband's premature ejaculation. The partners were encouraged to regularly practice the techniques discussed and come for review once a month.

sharing closeness, and focusing on mutual pleasure rather than on performance or technique. Boredom with a sexual routine may result in reduced desire and the couple will benefit from changes in positions or venues, or the addition of erotic materials. Vaginal lubricants can help moisten the vagina, reduce pain and discomfort, and improve arousal. Pelvic floor (Kegel) exercises can help with pain, arousal, and problems of orgasm: the patient is instructed to tighten the pelvic muscles as if stopping the stream of urine, hold for a count of five, relax and repeat the exercise several times a day. If dysfunction is present in the male partner, it is essential to treat it.

Step 9. Negotiate a treatment plan, compliance, participation, and responsibility

While the physician can help in excluding medical causes of sexual dysfunction,

---

BOX 12.3 MARITAL DISCORD AND SEXUAL PROBLEMS

A 44-year-old woman came to the hospital with her husband, with complaints of tiredness and pain in the limbs that was variable in onset and severity. Detailed and repeated physical examination and investigations ruled out the presence of a medical or psychiatric illness. On questioning the couple about their sex life, both complained about the minimal frequency of sex in their lives – about two or three times a year during the past 5 years. The patient was distressed by the lack of sex and stated that she felt unloved and uncared for. Whenever they did have sex, she was able to become aroused and reach orgasm. The woman and her husband held responsible jobs, and were stressed by work and household responsibilities. They were responsible and loving parents but most of the responsibility for the children's care fell on the patient as her husband was mostly away on business. It was evident that the patient did not suffer from a lack of desire; rather her poor sex life reflected stress, marital problems, and a reaction to her husband's lack of involvement.

The distress of both the partners was acknowledged and they were encouraged to talk about their difficulties, expectations of each other, and desires. This helped them to understand each other's needs as well as how the patient's physical symptoms and the couple's sexual problems were related to the difficulties in their relationship and emotional factors, rather than a physical illness. The couple was educated about normal sexuality and factors that can alter sexual functioning, including stress. The couple was advised to be more open in their communication with each other, regarding both day-to-day as well as sexual matters. They were asked to ensure that they spent more time with each other in leisure activities, such as going together to a movie or the park. The patient was asked to learn and regularly practice yoga and meditation to help reduce her anxiety and stress. Spending time in non-genital touching was encouraged and this provided the patient with some of the attention and affection that she needed. The couple was encouraged to practice the strategies discussed and come for review once a month.

BOX 12.4 OTHER FACTORS IN ETIOLOGY OF SEXUAL DYSFUNCTION

A number of other factors can be associated with a person's sexual dysfunction. These may be relevant to the etiology and may contribute to varying degrees. They may also be crucial in management. Some are listed below:

- *Partner Factors*
  - Partner's sexual problems
  - Partner's health status
- *Relationship Factors*
  - Poor communication
  - Discrepancies in desire for sexual activity
- *Individual Vulnerability Issues*
  - Poor body image
  - History of sexual abuse
  - History of emotional abuse
  - Psychiatric comorbidity (e.g. anxiety, depression)
  - Stressors (e.g. loss of employment, bereavement)
- *Cultural or Religious Factors*
  - Attitudes towards sexuality
  - Inhibitions to religious or cultural prohibitions against sexual activity/pleasure
- *Medical Concerns*
  - Medical comorbidity
  - Medication induced sexual dysfunction

BOX 12.5 COGNITION AND EMOTIONS RELATED TO SEXUAL DYSFUNCTION

Sexual response involves a complex interplay of physiology, emotions, experiences, beliefs, lifestyle, and relationships. Many women with sexual dysfunctions report a variety of contextual concerns, which affect their sexual function. Fear of pregnancy and infections, marital discord, substance use, emotional stress, and physical exhaustion contribute to dysfunction. The lack of erotic thoughts and disengagement thoughts during sexual activity are also common in women who report dysfunction. Sexual conservative beliefs seem to be closely related to hypoactive sexual desire and to arousal difficulties in some women. Body image beliefs and automatic thoughts focusing on self-body appearance seem to be associated with orgasmic disorder. Fear is a common predictor of vaginismus, while sadness, disillusion, guilt, and lack of pleasure and satisfaction are associated to hypoactive sexual desire. These issues need to be explored, discussed, and managed in therapy.

clarifying sexual misconceptions, suggesting simple techniques to improve function, and prescribing medication, the patient will have to implement the many suggestions for success. Consequently, there is a need to discuss patient participation and compliance with medication and offer psychological and sexual advice. Discuss with the patient the need to regularly practice the coping strategies and specific suggestions. Instill confidence in the patient and emphasize that many problems can be resolved with minor adjustments. Encourage the patient to take greater responsibility to improve her marital relationship, understand her own anxieties, and clarify them.

Step 10. Give a specific appointment for review

Regular review of progress is necessary for most patients and there should be scheduled, brief appointments every 2–4 weeks (i.e. avoiding "as-needed" appointments). These sessions should be utilized to assess the progress made and identify new difficulties. The physician's approach at these sessions should be that of a "cheer-leader" who provides encouragement and specific suggestions.

WILL I BE ABLE TO DO THIS IN MY BUSY CLINICAL PRACTICE?

The majority of people with sexual dysfunction require clarification of their misconceptions, education on normal sexual function, and simple advice on avoiding personal and other circumstances that cause difficulties. Simple suggestions, such as the use of vaginal lubricants and pelvic floor exercises, can help with pain, arousal, and problems of orgasm. The primary job of a physician is, therefore, to clarify issues, provide targeted solutions, and instill confidence in the patient. With practice, the efficiency of the technique used improves and such counseling can be used in real-life situations in a session of 10–15 minutes.

WHEN SHOULD I REFER A PATIENT FOR SPECIALIST HELP?

Sexual orientation or preference issues, severe marital discord, comorbid substance use or major psychiatric disorders, current or past abuse, or continued problems despite treatment in primary care may necessitate a psychiatric consultation. Uncontrolled diabetes or hypertension, medication-induced sexual dysfunction, or structural organic conditions may also need specialist intervention.

CONCLUSION

Sexual dysfunction in women is a problem that is rarely discussed, recognized, or managed in primary care. It is essential that the physician is comfortable discussing these issues with patients to allow for appropriate intervention and management.

13 Women's Mental Health

There are psychological issues that are unique to women, their social roles in life, and are also related to their reproductive physiological stages and cycles. These include premenstrual dysphoria, problems related to pregnancy and the postpartum period, and menopausal issues. Of particular significance are the problems that occur in pregnancy and the postpartum period as they not only affect the health of the woman, but also significantly influence the health of the child. In addition to physiological states, the mental health of women is significantly affected by the patriarchal society, with its subtle and not so subtle discrimination.

The management includes the elicitation of problems, understanding context, the provision of a safe and supportive environment, and prescribing medication, if necessary.

INTRODUCTION

Social and cultural factors such as societal attitudes to women, the multiple roles and expectations of them, and the unique stressors that they face play an important role in the mental health of women. In addition, biological factors that come into play at different times in the woman's life cycle also contribute to mental health difficulties.

This chapter discusses the diagnosis and management of problems specific to women that present in primary care and in general medical settings.

WHAT ARE THE COMMON PROBLEMS RELATED TO WOMEN THAT ARE SEEN IN PRIMARY CARE?

Common problems related to the menstrual cycle are premenstrual dysphoric symptoms and symptoms that occur during menopause. Low mood ("blues") during the postpartum period is common, while melancholic depression and psychosis are rare.

HOW DO WOMEN WHO ATTEND PRIMARY CARE MANIFEST SUCH PROBLEMS?

Though symptoms related to menstruation and menopause are widely prevalent, the fact that these can sometimes be severe and benefit from treatment is not common knowledge. As these issues are often considered embarrassing and something women are not encouraged to talk about, both physicians and patients are reluctant to discuss them. Many patients with such problems may present with physical symptoms, such as weakness, fatigue, aches and pains, or other medically unexplained physical symptoms.

As a result, these problems are often under-reported. Physicians may also play down their significance.

Symptoms of postpartum depression may often go unrecognized because the symptoms overlap with many of the usual discomforts of the puerperium (e.g. fatigue, pain, interrupted sleeping, and low libido). In addition, women are often reluctant to complain about their symptoms, perhaps because of perceived social expectations that new mothers are happy and should cope with the new responsibilities.

How common are these disorders in primary care?

While premenstrual discomfort is common, clinically significant symptoms causing impairment occur in 3%–8% of women of reproductive age. Postpartum blues are a transient but common condition and 30%–75% of women develop these mood changes, which resolve spontaneously. The prevalence of severe depression during the postpartum period is around 10% while that of postpartum psychosis has been reported as approximately 1–2 per 1000 live births.

What questions can I ask the patient to elicit her problems?

Before enquiring about clinical symptoms, it is essential to establish rapport with the patient and communicate a respectful and sensitive attitude to allow the woman to feel comfortable to discuss these issues. The language used must be simple and appropriate for the local culture. Providing privacy encourages disclosure. Open-ended questions, such as "Do you have any difficulties related to your menstrual cycle/following menopause?", "Do you experience changes in your mood associated with the menstrual cycle?", and "How have you been feeling after the birth of your baby?" will encourage the patient to talk about these problems. Questions to elicit psychotic symptoms are described in the chapter on psychosis.

What are the common causes of these disorders?

Psychiatric problems that occur in different stages of the reproductive cycle are considered multifactorial in origin with several contributing factors. These include genetic susceptibility which may be indicated by the presence of a family history of similar illness; hormonal changes including thyroid and reproductive hormones; and a multitude of environmental factors including stressors related to the multiple roles a woman has to handle, inadequate support from family and partner, financial difficulties, etc. In some cultures, with preference for boys, the birth of a baby girl is a cause of significant stress, marital and familial discord. In cultures with taboos about menstruation, there is increased stress during these periods for many women.

What happens to patients who do not get help from physicians?

Women with severe premenstrual and menopausal symptoms have difficulty carrying out their day-to-day functions secondary to their symptoms. Problems in the postpartum period can interfere with maternal–infant bonding and child development, can result in marital discord, and in severe cases is associated with a risk of suicide and infanticide.

How do these disorders present?

Premenstrual Syndrome and Dysphoria: These disorders are characterized by emotional and physical symptoms. The most common emotional symptom reported is mood swings; other symptoms include irritability, anxiety, a feeling of tension, sadness, increased sensitivity to rejection, and diminished interest in activities. These are usually accompanied by physical manifestations, which are abdominal bloating, headache, fatigue, and breast tenderness. Characteristically, there is an onset of symptoms with each cycle, with symptoms being most severe in the 4 days before menstruation, through the first 2–3 days of menses followed by a symptom-free period. Some women experience severe distress characterized by anger, irritability, and internal tension. These symptoms interfere with different aspects of the woman's life and functioning.

Postpartum Blues: This is a transient condition characterized by mild depressive symptoms, sadness, tearfulness, irritability, anxiety, insomnia, and decreased concentration. Symptoms develop within 2–3 days of delivery, peak over the next few days, and resolve spontaneously within two weeks.

Postpartum Depression: This condition typically emerges over the first 2–3 postpartum months but may occur at any point after delivery. The clinical manifestations of postpartum depression are similar to depression occurring at other times during a woman's life. Symptoms include sadness, reduced sleep (independent of that related to the baby's sleep habits), low energy, reduced appetite, weight, and libido. The patient may describe irritability, feelings of inadequacy and inability to care for the baby, anxiety, and guilt. When severe, patients may have suicidal or homicidal thoughts, aggressive behavior, psychotic features, and significantly impaired functioning.

Postpartum Psychosis: This condition, though rare, most commonly presents within two weeks of childbirth. Hallucinations and delusions are usually present along with disorganization of thought and bizarre behavior, similar to that described in the chapter on psychosis. Characteristic features in postpartum psychosis are associated symptoms of rapid mood changes, insomnia, anxiety, irritability, and agitation. Occasionally, the patient's mental status may fluctuate between periods of confusion and intermittent clearing without evidence of other causes of delirium. Postpartum psychosis may be associated with delusional beliefs that centre on the infant and auditory hallucinations that instruct the mother to harm herself or her infant, resulting in thoughts of suicide and/or homicidal ideation directed towards the infant and/or other children at home; therefore, it is considered a psychiatric emergency.

An episode of psychosis in the postpartum period may be a relapse or exacerbation of a pre-existing psychotic illness or bipolar disorder, or it may be the first episode of either illness. Women who have a bipolar disorder are at high risk of recurrence in pregnancy and postpartum.

Menopausal Symptoms: Natural menopause is the permanent cessation of menstrual periods, determined retrospectively after a woman has experienced 12 months of amenorrhea without any other obvious pathological or physiological cause usually occurring in the late forties to early fifties. Insomnia is a common symptom and may be present in association with hot flashes, anxiety, depression, or independently. There is a significant increased risk of new onset depression in women during the menopausal transition especially in those with a prior history of depression and fluctuations in reproductive hormone levels. Panic disorder may occur for the first time during menopause, or there may be a worsening of existing symptoms. Cognitive changes may occur secondary to anxiety and depression. A worsening of the course of schizophrenia and an exacerbation of mood symptoms in those with pre-exisitng psychosis and bipolar disorder is reported.

How should I proceed?

Once the syndrome is identified, a detailed history and clinical examination, including neurological, genital, and pelvic examinations, are essential in ruling out common medical problems that may present with such symptoms. Basic laboratory tests should be ordered (e.g. complete blood count, blood sugar levels, lipid levels, and serum creatinine), while special tests (e.g. thyroid function tests, prolactin, follicle-stimulating hormone, luteinizing hormone levels of human chorionic gonadotropin) may also be required. If there is suspicion of a cerebral event, such as cortical venous thrombosis, brain imaging should be considered. History of substance use and other medication use needs to be reviewed. Other psychological and social difficulties in the patient's life must be explored.

Common sources of stress include societal roles and expectations of women, patriarchal attitudes, and discrimination based on gender, which are common in many cultures. Disturbances in relationships with partner and other family members, obstetric events such as unplanned pregnancy, abortion, stillbirth, or neonatal death also contribute to mental ill health and distress. Problems in the areas of employment, finances, and health, difficulties balancing between the multiple roles and responsibilities expected of her, inadequate social support, physical and sexual abuse, and discrimination can produce significant distress and need to be understood and managed.

How do I manage patients with these problems?

It is essential to acknowledge the distress that the patient is experiencing. This encourages the patient to discuss their problems, conveys empathy, and provides reassurance. Discuss the patient's and family's concerns; an understanding of their perspectives on the problem will help to provide effective reassurance and education. Many women may be concerned that their mood changes related to periods may indicate a serious medical disorder; their misconceptions need clarification. Worries regarding anatomy and physiology may be present; self-esteem issues and concerns regarding their femininity may be present in women who have had an abortion, are menopausal, or have undergone genital surgery.

Given the cultural and religious taboos that exist regarding menstruation, patients need to be encouraged to freely discuss their worries. It is useful to educate the patient about symptoms that occur in a normal menstrual cycle, normal changes that occur as part of pregnancy, the postpartum period, and aging. Helping women to understand that many of their symptoms are normal and do not indicate pathology is useful. The stress of daily living, including concerns about work, family, and finances, can result in anxiety that worsens symptoms; helping the patient to understand the relationship between emotional factors and symptoms is also an important step. In the case of postpartum problems, the family should be specifically advised on the need to carefully supervise the patient and the baby, and the provision of adequate support to the mother.

MANAGEMENT

Premenstrual Disorders: The treatment goals for patients with premenstrual disorders are to relieve symptoms and improve functional impairment. Lifestyle measures such as regular exercise and stress reduction techniques are helpful. For women with moderate to severe symptoms, selective serotonin reuptake inhibitors (SSRIs) such as sertraline or fluoxetine may be useful (*see also* Chapter 23). These can be administered as a daily therapy or luteal phase-only treatment (starting on cycle day 14). If this does not help, oral contraceptive pills, estrogen, and progesterone may be tried in consultation with an obstetrician.

Postpartum Blues: These symptoms can be managed by providing reassurance and support for the woman. Providing adequate time for the patient to rest and sleep by involving other family members to help and care for the baby, especially at night, is essential. The blues usually resolve over two weeks. If symptoms persist or worsen, interventions for depression need to be considered.

Postpartum Depression: For patients with mild symptoms psychological support and intervention may be adequate, especially for lactating patients who want to avoid neonatal exposure to antidepressants. Encouraging the patient to do activities that give a sense of satisfaction and reduce the tendency to ruminate over negative thoughts is useful. Providing suggestions to help improve communication and problem-solving skills, and ensuring the involvement of the partner and other family members are helpful.

Patients with severe depression may have suicidal or homicidal behaviour, may be aggressive, and have psychotic features. They require close supervision and may need to be hospitalized. In addition to the psychological measures described above, such patients require antidepressant medication such as SSRIs (sertraline and paroxetine), serotonin-norepinephrine reuptake inhibitors, atypical antidepressants (bupropion or mirtazapine), and tricyclics (imipramine). The tricyclic agents and mirtazapine may be preferred when there is a need for sedation. For patients who do not respond to initial treatment with an antidepressant, referral to a psychiatrist is advisable so other options such as changing or augmenting antidepressant medication and electroconvulsive therapy (ECT) can be considered.

Postpartum Psychosis: Hospitalization is advised. Ensuring safety of the mother and the child is the immediate priority. Having the baby beside the mother is useful to facilitate bonding; however, the mother should not be left alone with the infant and the pair needs to be closely supervised. Antipsychotic medications are the treatment for psychosis and agitation in postpartum psychosis. These drugs need to be continued for up to two years after a single episode of psychosis. (*See also* Chapter 8 on Psychosis for details of drugs and dosages.) Careful monitoring of the mother and the child for adverse effects to antipsychotic medication is essential. Benzodiazepines in low doses may be necessary to reduce agitation initially; however, it should be avoided in breastfeeding mothers because of the risk of sedation to the child. ECT may be useful if a rapid response is needed to prevent harm, e.g. the woman is acutely agitated or at high risk for suicide or infanticide.

Postmenopausal Symptoms: Antidepressant medications such as SSRIs are useful in the treatment of postmenopausal symptoms. The usefulness of hormone replacement therapy is controversial. Educating women about what to expect during menopause decreases anxiety, depression, and irritability; a healthy, balanced diet, and regular exercise are thought to be helpful in diminishing the symptoms of depression.

USE OF PSYCHOTROPIC MEDICATION IN PREGNANCY AND LACTATION

The issues related to the use of psychotropic medication in pregnancy and lactation need to be discussed in detail with the patient and her family as there are risks and benefits that they need to be aware of before making an informed decision.

Pregnancy: Evidence is limited but available literature suggests that the risk of major congenital malformations varies among psychotropic medications with the greatest risk associated with valproate, carbamazepine, and lithium as compared to that with antipsychotics and antidepressants. Most studies have found that exposure during pregnancy to first- and second-generation antipsychotics does not appear to increase the risk of major physical malformations above rates observed in the general population. However, chronic administration of antipsychotics during the third trimester may cause symptoms of neonatal toxicity and withdrawal. Antenatal exposure to benzodiazepines appears to be associated with spontaneous abortion and preterm birth. Chronic administration of benzodiazepines proximal to delivery can cause neonatal toxicity and withdrawal. The risk of congenital abnormalities with lithium is low and may involve

---

BOX 13.1 PREMENSTRUAL DYSPHORIA

A 26-year-old college student presented with a long history of symptoms that had begun when she was in high school. About five days before the onset of menstruation, she described having uterine cramping, headache, breast tenderness, bloating, and constipation at which time she would become irritable, depressed, and prone to tears. These symptoms would reach a peak of intensity in three days and would result in her missing school or college for 1–2 days. The day her period began, the symptoms began to reduce.

A careful physical examination including a pelvic and breast examination was normal. There were no abnormalities evident on blood tests. The patient was educated about the nature of her difficulties and the possible reasons for her problems; her concerns regarding her symptoms were addressed. She was advised to reduce her intake of sugar and increase the fruit and vegetable in her diet; a regular exercise schedule was also begun. Sertraline 50 mg was commenced as a daily morning dose. By the second month, she reported an improvement and by the third month after beginning treatment, she was feeling much better and able to cope with the few symptoms that she had.

BOX 13.2 POSTPARTUM PSYCHOSIS

Ms A is a 27-year-old teacher who had delivered her first child seven days before the consultation. The pregnancy was planned and the birth eagerly awaited. She underwent an uncomplicated delivery, and her baby boy was full term and healthy. Three days after delivery, she told her mother that her husband was trying to poison her food and that her baby was staring at her strangely. She said she heard God speaking to her, commanding her to kill her baby so that all the other children in the world may prosper. In response to these hallucinations, she had attempted to strangle her child. She was able to sleep only for 2–3 hours at night, appeared preoccupied, and needed help to care for herself and the baby.

The patient was admitted to the hospital and kept under close supervision along with her baby. Physical examination including pelvic and neurological examinations were normal as were all the blood tests. The family was educated about the illness. Olanzapine was commenced at a dose of 5 mg and increased every 2–3 days to 15 mg a day. Breastfeeding was continued under close supervision. As she began to improve, she was encouraged to interact more with the baby and take on more tasks with respect to looking after the baby and herself. The patient's functioning and safety status was regularly reviewed. By the end of 10 days she was better and recovered fully within a period of three weeks. The family was discharged at the end of a month with advice to continue medication and regular follow-up.

BOX 13.3 PATHOLOGIZING NORMAL FUNCTION

While the American Psychiatric Association's Diagnostic and Statistical Manual 5 has a separate label and criteria called Premenstrual Dysphoric Disorder (PMDD), many scholars from psychology and social science disciplines have been critical of the category. They argue that such a disorder does not exist and women should not receive mental illness labels to seek help for their discomfort. They argue that the language of Premenstrual Syndrome (PMS) and PMDD is misleading and that its classification as a mental disorder stigmatizes women as mentally ill, covers up the social, economic, and structural causes for distress. They argue that emotional displays by men are considered normal, while those among women pathological. They suggest that such labels undermine women's self-esteem and feeds into stereotypes about women. They argue that these and other psychiatric diagnoses are mainly for the insurance and health industries so that physicians can claim reimbursements. They also open up the market for pharmaceutical solutions instead of focusing on the patriarchal culture and its negative impact on women.

the heart (e.g. Ebstein's anomaly of the tricuspid valve); second and third trimester lithium exposure can lead to neonatal complications and lithium toxicity. Valproate and carbamazepine are associated with spina bifida and craniofacial abnormalities.

Lactation: The nutritional, immunological, and psychological benefits of breastfeeding have been well documented. However, it is known that all psychotropic medications are transferred into breastmilk, and thus are passed on to the nursing infant. Therefore, the benefits of breastfeeding need to be weighed against risks to the infant for psychotropic medication.

Concentrations of psychotropic medication secreted in breast milk vary; the amount of medication to which an infant is exposed depends on several factors, including dosage of medication, rate of maternal drug metabolism, and frequency and timing of feedings. Therefore, exposure can be decreased by choosing medications with shorter half-lives, starting the drug at the lowest effective dose, avoiding the hind milk ejected during the second half of a feed (which is likely to have a higher concentration of maternal medication because of the higher lipid content). Restricting breastfeeding to times during which drug concentrations in breastmilk would be at their lowest levels or by taking medication immediately after breastfeeding is useful.

Most antidepressants are thought to be safe for use in breastfeeding women as there have been no reports of serious adverse events related to exposure to these medications. The exposure of infants to antipsychotics via human milk generally appears to be low and clinically insignificant. However, given the inadequate data available, breastfeeding is typically discouraged in patients treated with clozapine. Lithium is excreted at high levels in the mother's milk, and infant serum levels are relatively high, increasing the risk of neonatal toxicity; therefore, must be avoided, if possible. Exposure to carbamazepine and valproic acid in the breast milk has been associated with hepatotoxicity in the nursing infant.

The child must be carefully and regularly monitored for alertness, feeding, and weight gain. Behavioral changes, irritability, agitation, and excessive crying must be noted. In addition, infants should be assessed for known drug effects such as extra-pyramidal symptoms, constipation, and sedation in those exposed to antipsychotics. Additional caution about exposure through breastfeeding is warranted for premature, low birth weight, or sick infants. If adverse events in infants are suspected, mothers should immediately reduce or suspend breastfeeding.

CONCLUSION

Mental health problems related to women result from a complex interplay of psychological, social, and biological factors. These need to be dealt with in a sensitive manner and managed appropriately with psychosocial interventions. Women who are at risk for postpartum disorders because of a positive past history must be carefully monitored; risks and benefits regarding the medication must be discussed with the patient and family. Psychosocial interventions are of great benefit in this group of patients.

Section IV

Common Clinical Situations

14 Breaking Bad News

Physicians are frequently called upon to communicate unpleasant news related to diagnosis, treatment, and prognosis. Such disclosure has to be tailored to the needs of the individual and to the context. The steps in breaking bad news include assessment of the gap between the patient's expectation and reality, narrowing this gap, gently confirming the bad news, providing information, allowing the patient time to absorb the news and express emotions, clarifying doubts, making a joint management plan, and an appointment for review.

INTRODUCTION

Physicians, in their quest to alleviate illness and suffering, are constantly engaged in dealing with bad and tragic news. Breaking bad news, often an everyday event, mandates that the required skill is mastered by all who practice medicine. However, most medical schools and courses rarely teach the art of breaking bad news and let most budding physicians flounder and learn the skill at the expense of their patients. This chapter discusses the principles of and strategies for breaking bad news.

Bad news is defined as any news that drastically alters a person's view of his/her future. Estimating the gap between the patient's expectation of his/her situation and the reality of his/her condition is crucial. A large gap between expectation and reality suggests bad news. The key to breaking bad news is to establish the magnitude of the gap. The way a healthcare professional delivers bad news significantly influences the therapeutic relationship.

WHAT ARE THE COMMON SITUATIONS IN A MEDICAL SETTING THAT INVOLVE THE BREAKING OF BAD NEWS?

Common bad news situations can include informing a patient of a terminal disease, the recurrence of disease, the spread of disease, and the failure of treatment to alter the course and outcome of the disease. Other such situations include talking about the occurrence of irreversible adverse effects, results of genetic tests, or the issue of palliative care and resuscitation. Some examples are: a patient who has been diagnosed to have cancer, a patient who has been told he/she is HIV-positive, or a couple who is told they cannot have children.

WHAT ARE THE MODELS FOR BREAKING BAD NEWS?

There are three general models for breaking bad news: (i) the non-disclosure model; (ii) the full disclosure model; and (iii) the individualized disclosure model. The non-disclosure model, as the name suggests, does not allow the physician to discuss the bad news or its implications and keeps the patient and his/her family in the dark. This model is untenable as it provides false hope, denies the patient an opportunity to come to terms with his/her situation, undermines the doctor–patient relationship, precludes the patient's participation in his/her own treatment, creates barriers within the family unit, and obstructs vital mutual support.

At the other end of the spectrum is the full disclosure model, in which the physician explains all details of the situation in one sitting without assessing its impact on the patient and his/her family. This model is paternalistic and does not take into account the amount of information given and the timing of the disclosure, and hence, may not be appropriate for all patients.

The individualized disclosure model takes into consideration the varying needs of patients in terms of their capacity to cope and the amount of information they want. It allows the patient time to absorb and adjust to the bad news, builds confidence in the doctor–patient relationship, and forms the basis of mutual decision-making.

WHAT IS THE PROCESS OF INDIVIDUALIZED DISCLOSURE?

Often, the task of breaking bad news is much easier than expected, as many patients with serious medical conditions suspect the diagnosis. Their suspicions and doubts are often based on the magnitude and complexity of diagnostic testing, and the behavior and silence of the doctors, nurses, technicians, and members of their own family. In such subjects, the doctor needs to confirm the views that the patient may already hold.

On the other hand, the task is more difficult when the patient and the family have not considered the possibility of grave prognosis, i.e. of bad news. In such situations, the task will need to be addressed in small steps, with a gradual progression, giving the patient time to handle the new information.

The process of individualized disclosure, as the name implies, tailors the task of providing bad news and information to the patient's context, personality, and views. The breaking of bad news requires some preparation. Review the patient's condition, reports, basic prognosis, and treatments before starting the session of breaking bad news. Plan what to say and ensure adequate time for the interview. The interview should be conducted in a private setting, avoiding interruptions such as the phone. The patient should also be given the option of bringing in confidants to discuss issues.

The task can be divided into manageable steps, as listed below:

- find out what the patient already knows or suspects
- assess the gap between the patient's expectations and the reality
- find out how much the patient wants to know
- provide information
- allow the patient time to absorb the information
- encourage the patient to express his feelings
- clarify any doubts, misconceptions, and fears
- briefly state the management plan in simple language
- provide details if the patient wants to know
- state that you are available for further clarification.

Find out what the patient already knows or suspects

The first step in breaking bad news is to find out what the patient knows. Simply reiterating the current situation and asking the patient for his or her opinion on the problem can obtain this information. For example, "The pain has been worsening for some weeks. Do you have any ideas as to the nature of your illness?" Alternatively, ask "What have you already been told about your illness?"

Such reiteration of the situation or directly asking the patient what he/she already knows about the disease is a good starting point to assess how much information the patient already has and what he/she suspects are the underlying problems and issues.

Assess the gap between the patient's expectation and the reality

Assess the gap between the patient's expectations and the reality. If the gap between expectation and reality is narrow, the task of breaking bad news is easier than expected. Many patients with serious medical conditions suspect the possible diagnosis. In such subjects, the doctor needs to gently confirm views that the patient may already hold. For example, "The biopsy report confirms our suspicions of cancer."

If the gap between expectation and reality is wide, the task is more difficult. Give a warning that things are not as good as one hoped they might have been. For example, "The biopsy report is not as good as we had hoped."

Find out how much the patient wants to know

The process of individualized disclosure demands that the patient's needs and wishes be respected. This necessitates that the physician periodically asks permission to provide more details or to proceed with the treatment plan. Such individualized disclosure implies that the patient's point of view will be valued and followed. For example, "Would you like to know the details of the illness or would you prefer that we make a plan and get on with it?" This model also suggests that there is no right answer or specific approach and that the patient may choose the options he/she wants.

Provide information

If the patient clearly indicates that he/she is interested, proceed to give information in small chunks and in a stepwise manner. Use simple language that is understandable to lay people. It is more important to communicate the seriousness of the condition and talk about its treatment than to mention technical terms. For example, "The biopsy suggests that the lump is not benign. It is a form of cancer." Discussing the pathology in simple language is useful. Drawing simple diagrams to explain medical or surgical procedures will improve the patient's understanding of the issues and will prepare him/her for the investigations and interventions.

Allow the patient time to absorb the information

Bad news, by definition, may alter the course of a person's life. It may have serious implications on health, family, work, finances, and life. Ensure long pauses between pieces of information in order that the person is able to absorb and understand the magnitude of the problem and its implications. This is necessary so that the patient and his family have time to soak up the significance of the new information.

Encourage the patient to express his feelings

The communication of new information and bad news usually has a major impact on the person and his/her life and family. Such sudden change in direction results in many emotions, often not pleasant. Encouraging patients to express their feelings is essential for the physician to assess the nature of the impact of the new information and bad news. It will allow the physician to decide on how to proceed with the session. For example, "The diagnosis must have come as a shock to you and I can see that you are upset; it would be upsetting for anyone."

It is important to discuss the patient's feelings and express understanding and respect for them, in addition to discussing the implications of the bad news. It is also important to permit the patient to be distressed and express it without feeling bad about it. Explaining that such emotions are normal in the context of the stressful situation will allow the patient to ventilate her/his concerns.

Clarify any doubts, misconceptions, and fears

Bad news related to health and disease is often difficult for patients to understand. The technical terms, the complex interventions, the cost, and the implications would confuse any normal and competent human being. Giving permission to ask questions and clarifying doubts is crucial for a realistic understanding of the problem. Diseases such as cancer, HIV, and tuberculosis are dreaded conditions, and many lay people diagnosed with them may have misconceptions about the disease, its treatment, and prognosis. Identifying fears and clarifying misconceptions, which contribute to such apprehensions, will go a long way in alleviating psychological distress and in improving coping. For example, "I realize that it is difficult for you to accept the diagnosis. Would you like any clarification?", "Cancer is often considered a fatal illness. However, there are many varieties of cancer, many new medications, and when identified at an early stage can lead to a good outcome. Do you have any concerns which you might want to discuss?"

Repetition of the facts may sometimes be required because of the patient's emotional distress, the technical nature of the medical interventions involved, or because the patient does not remember the information previously given.

Briefly state the management plan

Briefly stating the management plan will allow the physician to orient the patient to the next phase of therapy. The individualized disclosure model mandates that the physician seek the patient's permission to provide details. While some people would like to know all the details of the procedures and therapy, others prefer that the doctor makes a plan and carries it through. Explaining the procedures, treatments, schedules, and cost in simple language is mandatory. Providing details for those who specifically request them is also part of good medical care.

The treatment schedule should be explained in a systematic manner. For example,

"We plan to give you strong medicines to treat the cancer. Though the treatment will make you sick, it is worth it as the chances of remission are good."

Provide further details if the patient wants to know

The opportunity to discuss the implications in greater depth should always be provided. Assessing the individual's needs for information, providing necessary information, and managing the disclosure in a stepwise manner is crucial. For example, "This is overwhelming, isn't it? It must be a worrying time. Do you have any doubts or need any clarification?" The provision of detailed information to those who specifically seek it will also mandate that the physician takes responsibility to provide it in a sensitive fashion, allowing the patient and his/her family to understand, handle, and cope with the information. It is also important to assess the patient's readiness and know when to stop.

State that you are available for further clarification

Give a definite appointment to the patient and relatives for reviewing the situation, for providing more information, and for clarifying doubts and fears. The patient should also be given the option of bringing family members and confidants for reviews so that the family's doubts and misconceptions can be clarified. The advantage of including family members in treatment is obvious as they can provide continuous support – physical, emotional, and financial.

HOW DO I ANSWER QUERIES REGARDING THE SUCCESS OF TREATMENT?

Patients often like to know the chances of success of various therapies. Such questions are difficult to answer using figures. For example, it may be difficult to explain to an individual patient his chances of remission for a treatment, which has a 90% chance of success. Although the general perspective on recovery should be mentioned, the central attitude should be one of "prepare for the worst and hope for the best".

It may be better to acknowledge the state of uncertainty, which, though unpleasant, does not offer false hope. Supporting the patient and family through such uncertainty is crucial.

HOW DO I RESPOND WHEN PATIENTS SEEK ADVICE ON MAKING PERSONAL DECISIONS?

The sudden changes in risks related to survival in patients with cancer and HIV raise a whole host of personal decisions related to life, work, family, finances, and property. It is better not to make decisions for patients. Such decisions are best postponed until the choices become clear to the patient and the family. The task of those counseling patients is to present the facts, and the patients and their families make their own decisions.

WHAT DO I DO IF THE PATIENT'S RELATIVES DO NOT WANT THE PATIENT TO BE TOLD THE DIAGNOSIS?

Sometimes the patient's relatives feel that the patient should not be told about a diagnosis such as cancer. It is useful to mention that many patients with cancer and other grave illnesses usually guess the seriousness of the condition, but feel isolated as everybody around them avoids the issue. The strain of deceiving the patient is also enormous. Relatives should be advised that if the patient gives a clear signal that he/she wants to know about his/her illness, they should talk about it rather than worsen the distress by avoiding the subject.

WHAT DO I DO IF THE PATIENT BEGINS TO CRY WHEN I AM TALKING?

In general, it is better to wait for the person to stop crying. You could otherwise acknowledge it and suggest: "Would you like to take a break now until you are ready to start again?" Appear calm and remember that tears are not an emergency that must be stopped. Most patients are somewhat embarrassed if they begin to cry and will not continue for long.

CONCLUSION

Breaking bad news is part of being a doctor and is a part of every physician's daily routine and practice. The ability to break bad news is essential for good medical practice. The steps described provide a simple systematic guide. Simple details lie between success and failure. The issues discussed are guidelines, not rules. These are possible choices and alternatives, which can be used in busy medical and surgical settings in real-life situations. Even long interviews do not last more than 10–15

BOX 14.1   COMMUNICATING DIAGNOSIS, TREATMENT PLANS, AND PROGNOSIS

Medicine, in keeping with its status in society, always had a paternalistic culture. Doctors listened to patients' concerns, examined them, ordered laboratory investigations, diagnosed disease, prescribed medication, and prognosticated about course and outcome. While they did explain the issues to their patients, medical perspectives and opinions guided their decisions. Patients were expected to follow their advice. The prevalent paternalistic culture within the medical profession often dismissed patient perspectives and did not take kindly to objections or different points of view. The culture within the profession complicated issues by dismissing individual's rights of self-determination as inconsequential to the science of cure.

The gradual shift from the paternalistic model to a contractual relationship between patients and physicians was an important milestone. The established philosophical tradition argued that knowledge is always good in itself and to remain ignorant deprives people of their choice and consequently of their autonomy. Freedom, dignity, truth-telling, promise-keeping, and justice became central to the relationship. The individual's "right to know" undergirded the contractual model. Informed consent became standard.

BOX 14.2 INFORMED CONSENT

The concept of informed consent was based on the moral and legal principles and arguments of patient autonomy. It demanded disclosure of information from doctors and intellectual capacity and voluntary decisions from patients. Competence or decision-making capacity includes the ability to understand the options and their consequences, evaluate the personal costs and benefits of each alternative, and to relate them to one's own values and priorities.

Informed consent necessitates that information be provided in a language that is easily understood by patients to be able to make autonomous decisions. The amount of information transmitted should be enough for a reasonable person to make decisions. The disclosure should include possible benefits and risks and the probabilities of their occurrence. The selection of the clinical option related to diagnosis and treatment has to be voluntary, i.e. without coercion or influence. The process also involves the patient giving permission to pursue the chosen alternative. Patient-centered approaches also mandate considerations of the cultural context.

BOX 14.3 THE SIX-STEP SPIKES* MODEL TO CLARIFY DIAGNOSIS AND PROGNOSIS

1. Setting – Getting started
2. Perception – What does the patient want to know?
3. Invitation – How much does the patient want to know?
4. Knowledge – Share the information.
5. Emotion – Respond to feelings.
6. Subsequent – Plan next steps and follow up.

* Baile WF, Buckman R, Lenzi R, Glober G, Beale EA, Kudelka AP. SPIKES – A six-step protocol for delivering bad news: Application to the patient with cancer. Oncologist. 2000; 5: 302–311.

minutes. All health professionals – doctors, nurses, social workers, and counselors – can use them.

Breaking bad news is difficult. However, it is part of the job of physicians involved in patient care. The technique of breaking bad news is crucial for those directly involved in the clinical decision-making process. It involves helping the patient and family understand the condition, providing support, and minimizing the risk of overwhelming distress or prolonged denial. Doing it well can facilitate adaptation to the illness and strengthen the doctor–patient relationship. The required skills can be mastered with practice. Such expertise will improve the quality of patient care.

15 The Angry or Tearful Patient

Physicians often encounter angry or tearful patients and relatives in their practice. The steps in management include acknowledging the emotion, exploring the reasons, giving permission to express feelings, admitting responsibility, and apologizing if the grievance is genuine, shifting the focus from the issue to the person, allowing the subject to explain the situation, and making a plan to tackle the issues.

INTRODUCTION

While physicians are professionals who have to manage a variety of patients and tolerate diverse behaviors, they routinely encounter patients who experience emotions and demonstrate behaviors that interfere with their care. Their behaviors evoke negative feelings and responses from health professionals. Such negative reactions make health professionals averse to interacting with these so-called "difficult" patients. For example, patients who are angry can make the doctor defensive, avoid discussing issues, reduce the time for interaction, make their physicians take a superficial approach to care, or even refuse treatment. Many emotional reactions and behaviors of patients can result in aversive reactions from healthcare professionals: sadness and depression, fear and anxiety, excessive dependency, competitiveness and challenging behavior, narcissism, passive aggression, and treatment refusal.

Nevertheless, a careful reading of these situations suggests that physicians are often unprepared and not adequately trained to manage such situations. Consequently, they blame patients for these behaviors and assume that it is not part of their duty to manage them. This chapter discusses simple strategies to recognize and manage difficult patients. The use of these principles results in a reduction of patient distress and physician unease.

Occasionally, patients and their relatives are also upset by hospital policies. They may be troubled by institutional procedures. Often they are distressed by the way the hospital staff have treated them or their relatives. They can become angry. They can also become sad and tearful because of their circumstances, diagnosis, treatment, or prognosis (Box 15.1). These situations occur frequently in busy medical and surgical settings in general hospitals. Rarely does the medical curriculum prepare physicians in the management of these complex situations. This chapter discusses the principles and steps in handling such circumstances.

The "difficult" patient can be managed using some basic steps (Box 15.2).

BOX 15.1 STEPS IN MANAGING ANGRY OR TEARFUL PATIENTS

1. Acknowledge the emotion
2. Explore the reasons
3. Encourage expression of feelings
4. Admit responsibility and apologize if the grievance is genuine
5. Shift focus from the issue to the person
6. Allow the subject to explain the situation
7. Make a plan to tackle the issues

MANAGING AN ANGRY SUBJECT

Busy hospital settings are stressful for patients, relatives, and for the hospital staff. The stress of these settings is because bad news and crises are ever-present. The staff is often overworked, thus straining many doctor–patient interactions. The patients and their relatives can become angry about hospital policies or procedures or due to specific interaction with the staff. Managing an angry or irritable patient or relative is a delicate task. Such situations require tact. The frequency of such occurrences demands the need for some training in their management.

The principles of managing such subjects include the acknowledgment of the emotion, exploring causation, encouraging the subject to express the angst, admitting responsibility if the grievance is genuine, shifting focus from the issue to the person, allowing the person to ventilate the anger, and making a plan to tackle the issues. Examples for each step are given in Box 15.3. These steps in management also allow for reflection of the person's emotion, legitimizing their concerns. These provide support, demonstrate respect for the individual, and build partnerships between physician and the patient.

Acknowledging anger and encouraging the person to express it are important first steps. Avoiding the emotion is like ignoring the elephant in the room. Being defensive

BOX 15.2 EMOTIONAL REACTIONS AND BEHAVIORS OF "DIFFICULT" PATIENTS

- Sadness and depression
- Fear and anxiety
- Excessive dependency
- Competitiveness and challenging behavior
- Narcissism
- Passive-aggression
- Treatment refusal

**BOX 15.3   EXAMPLES FOR STEPS IN THE MANAGEMENT OF AN
            ANGRY SUBJECT**

1. Acknowledge the emotions
   Example: "I can see that you are angry and upset."

2. Explore the reasons for such emotions
   Example: "Tell me what has upset you? Tell me about the problems you are facing."

3. Encourage the person to express his/her feelings
   Example: "I can see that you have reason to feel this way."

4. Admit responsibility and apologize if the grievance is genuine
   Example: "I am sorry. I did not realize that you had to wait so long to be seen."

5. Shift the focus from the issue to the person
   Example: "It must be difficult for you to see your relative in pain."

6. Allow the subject to explain the situation
   Example: "Tell me the details and I will try to help."

7. Make a plan to tackle the issues
   Example: "I will give you a specific appointment for your next visit so that you will not have to wait."

---

about the situation may exacerbate the problem as the subject's reaction may be justified. Criticizing the subject without finding out his/her point of view is usually disastrous. Similarly, defending colleagues, hospital policies, or procedures without finding out the circumstances will usually make things worse. Showing concern is cardinal to resolving the situation. Seeing the issues from the other person's perspective is often helpful. Putting oneself in their shoes will go a long way in providing an empathetic response. Resolution of such conflict is mandatory for the provision of compassionate care to people who have a variety of diseases and may be facing different degrees of crisis and stress. The provision of psychological support is a part of the job of a physician and health professional.

Managing a tearful subject

Sadness, depression, and tears are commonly seen in situations in which bad news is communicated, making hospitals a common setting for such presentations. Patients and their relatives, often overwhelmed by bad news and weighed down by the health crisis, can become tearful. Many physicians become uncomfortable with the show of such emotions. With a little practice, they can manage the situation and resolve what looks like a major embarrassment.

The steps in managing a tearful person are similar to those employed to defuse anger. The steps include acknowledging distress, encouraging the person to express sorrow, finding out the extent of the suffering and anguish, shifting the focus from the

BOX 15.4   EXAMPLES FOR STEPS IN THE MANAGEMENT OF A TEARFUL PATIENT

1. Acknowledge the emotion
   Example: "I can see that you are upset."

2. Explore the reasons for such emotion
   Example: "Tell me what has upset you" or "Tell me about the problems you are facing."

3. Encourage the person to express his/her feelings
   Example: "I can see that you have reason to feel this way."

4. Admit responsibility and apologize if the grievance is genuine
   Example: "I am sorry. I did not realize that the side-effects were so incapacitating."

5. Shift the focus from the issue to the person
   Example: "It must be difficult for you to cope with the symptoms, the adverse effects of the treatment, and also with work and family. It would be difficult for anybody."

6. Allow the subject to explain the situation
   Example: "Tell me the details and we can see how each of these issues can be managed."

7. Make a plan to tackle the issues
   Example: "We can discuss the issues with your wife. Can you bring her along when you come for the next appointment?"

issue to the person, showing concern, and making a plan to tackle the issues. Examples of how to manage such patients and their relatives are briefly given in Box 15.4.

CONCLUSION

Angry and tearful people are often encountered in the hospital setting. Learning to manage such people and situations is part of a doctor's job. The general principles in the management of "difficult" patients include manifesting empathy, acknowledging distress, exploring context, admitting responsibility for procedural lacunae, if any, shifting focus to person, and making a plan to mange issues.

Managing the so-called "difficult" patients should be part of the medical curriculum and training for physicians. Understanding the principles will allow for mastery and will add to the repertoire of doctors.

These principles and steps allow physicians to move towards a person and patient-centered approach to care. Small details separate success from disaster. Mastering the technique is only a matter of practice. The ability to diffuse such situations is helpful for patients and their relatives, and can be a source of satisfaction for physicians.

16 The Disturbed and Violent Patient

Although many people believe that people with mental illness are violent, the evidence suggests otherwise. Nevertheless, violent and disturbed patients are occasionally brought to general medical settings. The urgency of such situations requires that physicians understand the issues involved in their management. The steps in diagnosis include assessing the severity of the violence, the exclusion of paranoid psychosis, organic and medical causes, and substance use. The management of violence includes the use of restraints and psychotropic medication to calm the person. Communication and counseling are also important ingredients. Specific techniques are detailed.

INTRODUCTION

Many people tend to believe that people with mental illness are violent. However, the evidence argues otherwise (Box 16.1). However, a minority of people with mental illness can exhibit violence. General physicians are occasionally called to manage such patients.

The management of people who are violent and disturbed requires skill and teamwork. It requires quick yet comprehensive assessments with a focus on safety of both the patient and the hospital staff. The patient's aggression and violence need to be controlled quickly. It requires verbal skill so that the person is safely restrained with a minimal amount of force. Teamwork and coordination between physicians, nurses, and hospital staff is paramount. This chapter briefly discusses the issues related to managing violence in the hospital setting (Box 16.2).

WHAT ARE THE CAUSES OF VIOLENCE?

The causes of violence seen in hospital settings differ from those seen in other situations. While the police usually manage violent people with antisocial personality, people with mental illness who are violent are brought to emergency departments of hospitals. The referral pathways are usually able to discern differences; even when the police is called to restrain people with mental illness who are violent, they often recognize the fact that such people need medical help.

The causes of violence and extreme aggression among people with mental illness are many (Table 16.1). Organic and medical conditions, which produce intracranial pathology, can cause delirium and seizures, which can result in violence. People with substance dependence, intoxication, and withdrawal can become violent, particularly

BOX 16.1   MENTAL ILLNESS AND VIOLENCE

- The belief that people with mental illness are violent is not based on evidence; it is a myth created by the media.
- The link between violence and mental illness is weak; mental illness is neither necessary nor sufficient to cause violence.
- The vast majority of people with mental illness are not violent. In fact, people with mental illness are at a greater risk of hurting themselves or being hurt by others.
- Most of the predictors of violence are sociodemographic and economic (e.g. young, male, single, and from lower socioeconomic status).
- Substance abuse is a major determinant of violence independently. When it occurs concurrently with mental illness, it requires early intervention programs for substance dependence.
- Violence can occur in a minority of people with mental illness when a constellation of factors including the following combine: young, male, single, drug abuse, first episode, and untreated psychosis
- Violence, when occasionally seen, is often due to frightening visual and auditory hallucinations and paranoid and persecutory delusional beliefs.
- The public tends to exaggerate strength of the association between mental illness and violence and their own personal risk.

BOX 16.2   PUBLIC PERCEPTION OF VIOLENCE AND MENTAL ILLNESS

- Probability of violence among people with mental illness is universally over-estimated.
- Public perceptions of the link between mental illness and violence is central to stigma and discrimination of people with mental illness.
- Such public perception means that the general population is more likely to condone forced legal action and coerced treatment when violence is an issue.
- The presumption of violence may also provide a justification for bullying and victimizing people with mental illness.
- High rates of victimization among people with mental illness often go unnoticed by clinicians and undocumented in the clinical record.

when these are associated with delirium and psychosis. Those with mental illness (schizophrenia, mania, delusional disorders, and psychotic depression) can also present with markedly disturbed behavior and violence. People with personality disorders are at a higher risk of violence.

TABLE 16.1

Common Causes of Violence in Hospital Settings

- Organic Mental Disorders
    - *Seizures:* Complex partial; can also occur in pre- and post-ictal periods of other types
    - *Intracranial pathology:* Trauma (recent, old), infection, neoplasms, cerebrovascular accidents, degenerative diseases
    - *Systemic disorders:* Disorders that cause delirium
    - *Substance use:* Alcohol, cocaine, amphetamines, withdrawal from benzodiazepines
    - *Medication-related:* Steroid and anticholinergic drugs
- Functional Psychoses
    - schizophrenia
    - delusional disorder
    - mania
    - psychotic depression
- Non-psychotic, Non-organic Disorders
    - personality disorders

WHAT ARE THE PRINCIPLES OF THE MANAGEMENT OF VIOLENCE?

The two principles include the assessment of the severity of the violence and the evaluation of possible psychopathology with a view to assessing its predictability.

WHAT ARE THE STEPS IN THE ASSESSMENT OF VIOLENCE?

1. Assess the severity of the violence
2. Evaluate the evidence for diagnosis
    - Exclude paranoid delusions
    - Exclude organic and medical causes
    - Exclude substance use
    - Exclude psychosis
    - Attempt to establish the diagnosis

Both these steps have to be undertaken quickly, often immediately on arrival on the scene. While the challenge appears daunting, it can be mastered with practice.

Step 1. Assessing the severity of violence

The first step is to assess the nature and severity of the violence. The patient's history, behavior, and surroundings are used to gauge violence. Injuries to the patient and onlookers, damage to property, and the amount of force required to restrain the patient are pointers to the magnitude of the violence. Increased severity of violence demands greater caution. The assessment of severity is usually made on reaching the scene, with a quick glance at the patient and those around him/her.

Step 2. Evaluate the evidence for cause/diagnosis

The second step is to attempt to evaluate the evidence to establish the diagnosis or the cause of violence. The urgency of the situation usually does not permit a detailed history and examination, which are practiced during a routine clinical assessment. However, general questions have to be answered, broad categories assessed and excluded, and a tentative diagnosis made. A simple decision-tree is shown in Figure 16.1.

After the assessment of the magnitude of the violence, the next step in management is to make a tentative diagnosis. A brief history will suggest or exclude the possibilities of paranoid presentations with persecutory beliefs, organic and medical causes, substance intoxication, and psychosis.

Paranoid and persecutory beliefs can be symptoms of organic psychoses, substance dependence, and functional mental disorders. Individuals with such firmly held convictions that people are trying to harm/kill them are usually very scared, and will misinterpret even the most innocuous and neutral stimuli and generalize their delusional beliefs to include the doctor and hospital staff. Usually violence seen in hospital settings is due to persecutory delusions. Such patients may have acted on their paranoid beliefs, quarreled with relatives and neighbors, and may have abused and assaulted them. The

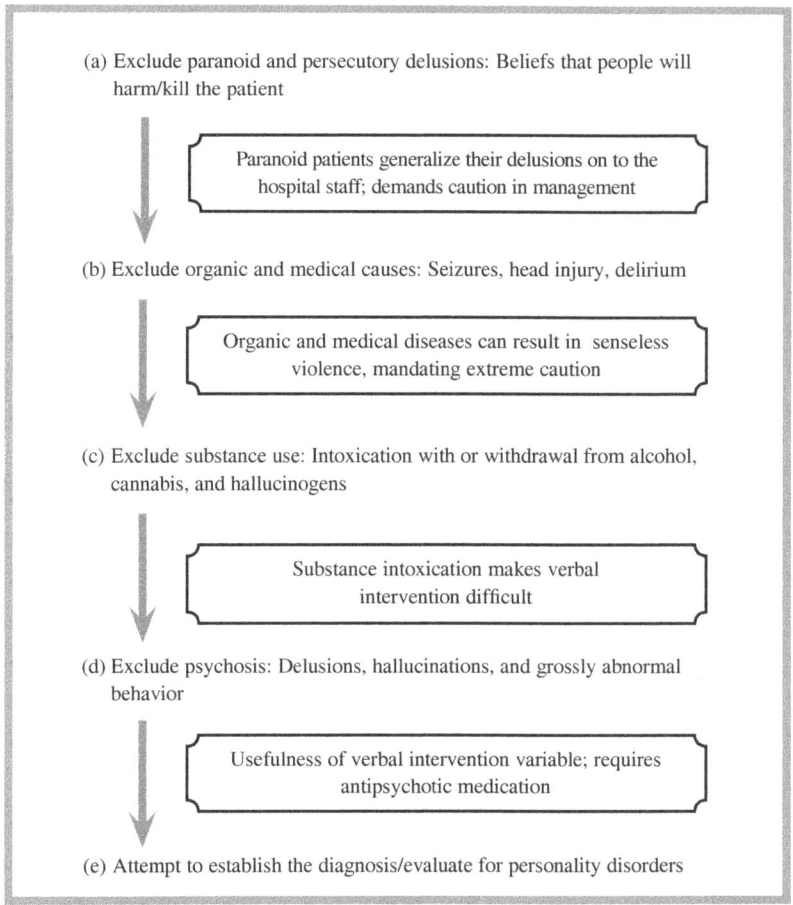

Figure 16.1 A simple decision tree to evaluate causes of violence/clinical diagnosis

relatives, in their attempts to restrain the patient, would have retaliated. After such assault, patients are usually brought to hospital. The number of people accompanying the patient, the state of their clothes (e.g. torn, bloodied, etc.), and their behavior towards the patient will give an indication of the magnitude and dangerousness of the violence.

A quick screening for organic violence is mandatory. A history of head injury, seizures, loss of consciousness, fever, and acute confusional states has to be excluded. Such medical conditions can result in senseless and unprovoked violence; in such situations, verbal intervention may not be successful and the person will need medication and physical restraint.

An assessment of behavior and speech, in addition to a brief enquiry, will elicit the use of substances and possible intoxication and withdrawal. Alcohol, cannabis, cocaine, and hallucinogen intoxication can result in violence. Patients who are intoxicated may be difficult to control using verbal commands; they may require medication and may need to be physically restrained.

A history to suggest strange beliefs, auditory and visual hallucinations, and grossly abnormal behavior would support the possibility of a psychosis. The presence of a cheerful or irritable mood with expansive ideas and hyperactivity suggests mania. A diagnosis of mania does provide some confidence; such patients do not resort to violence unless provoked.

The absence of psychosis would suggest a diagnosis of personality disorder. Patients with antisocial and borderline personalities can present occasionally to hospital with violence. More commonly, people with antisocial personalities often land up with the police rather than in the hospital. However, a diagnosis of personality disorder suggests that they can be talked out of violence.

The clinician can buy time by agreeing to some of the patient's demands until hospital staff arrives in numbers large enough to physically restrain the patient.

WHAT ARE THE GENERAL INTERVENTIONS TO MANAGE VIOLENCE?

Although the preceding discussion emphasized the need to make a diagnosis, most patients can be managed without reaching a definitive conclusion about the cause of violence or the exact medical or psychiatric diagnosis. Some general strategies are given in Table 16.2.

Intervention strategies, though focused on patient management and care, necessarily have to take into account the protection of the attending hospital staff. The examination area should provide some privacy but should not be isolated. It should have heavy furniture, which cannot be easily moved, and should not have objects that can be thrown or used as missiles. The physical distance between the patient and the doctor is important. While the doctor should be close to the individual to facilitate conversation, it is prudent to stay an arm's length away. The staff should also be ready to intervene to prevent assault and injury.

Although the management of violence is stressful for hospital staff, a calm appearance helps reduce the intensity of emotions in the patient. Similarly, intense eye contact and loud or aggressive speech aggravate the already tense situation and

---

TABLE 16.2

General Strategies to Manage Violence

1. Physical setting:
   − Remove objects that can be used as missiles/thrown.

2. Appearance:
   − Present a calm exterior.
   − Show concern and respect for the patient and his/her views.

3. Eye contact:
   − Avoid intense eye contact.

4. Speech:
   − Speech should be soft, non-judgmental, non-provocative, neutral, and concrete.
   − Listen to the patient; facilitate speech.

5. Verbal interaction:
   − Avoid premature interpretations.
   − Avoid making promises that cannot be kept.
   − Use "counterprojective techniques", e.g. "Who is troubling you?"

6. Physical intervention:
   − Physical restraint when the possibility of injury is imminent.

7. Precautions against physical assault:
   − Keep a distance of more than an arm's length from the patient.
   − Stand sideways with arms ready for self-defense.
   − Be prepared for sudden assault.
   − Observe the patient's movements carefully.
   − Stand or sit next to the exit.
   − Play for time if weapons are present.
   − Leave the room if you suspect that there may be concealed weapons.

8. Measures to restrict injury if assaulted:
   − If grabbed, gain immediate control of the grabbing hand.
   − If bitten, push bitten part inside the patient's mouth and close his/her nostrils.
   − If choked, tuck your chin in to protect your trachea and blood vessels.
   − If pushed to the floor, place your feet towards the patient to block further assault.

---

should be avoided. Statements aimed at preventing the generalization of persecutory beliefs are often helpful, as they tend to direct the patient's attention away from the attending staff. For example, "Tell me who are the people who are trying to harm you?" is a "counterprojective technique", which should be employed as it forces the patient to consider the staff on their side rather than against them, thus preventing the generalization of their paranoid beliefs. Such statements also provide a greater chance of establishing a rapport with people who are disturbed.

While it is difficult to predict assaults, it is mandatory to recognize a rise in tension, and every attempt must be made to reduce and defuse it. Verbal interventions should be attempted in all people who are disturbed and violent, although those who present with severe violence may require physical restraints.

The commands to initiate action, control and physically restrain patients should be rehearsed so that they can be efficiently employed when the situation arises. At least five people are necessary to restrain an individual, with each taking control of a limb and one person controlling the head. The simplest restraint is one where the patient is made to lie supine and the limbs are restrained (i.e. tied to the bed). Close and regular monitoring of the vital signs of all patients who are restrained is mandatory (e.g. every half hour). Every precaution should be taken to prevent injury to the patient. The use of cotton pads to prevent ischemic compression of the limbs is useful.

The physician dealing with such situations should have leadership qualities and members of the "emergency team" need to be knowledgeable regarding the management of violent patients. In addition, strategies to be used in different situations require regular rehearsal and updating.

WHAT PSYCHOTROPIC MEDICATION IS USED TO CONTROL VIOLENT PATIENTS?

The main classes of psychotropics used to control violent patients are antipsychotics and benzodiazepines (Table 16.3). Antipsychotics are used when the violence is secondary to psychotic disorders. The route of administration depends on the urgency

TABLE 16.3

Recommended Medications, Route of Administration, Dose, and Schedule

Drug	Dose	Route	Schedule	Maximum dose/day
Antipsychotic medication				
Olanzapine	10 mg	Oral	Repeated after few hours	20 mg/day
	10 mg	IM	(should not be administered along with IM benzodiazepines)	
Chlorpromazine	100–200 mg	Oral	Repeated every 2–4 hours	600 mg/day
Haloperidol + promethazine hydrochloride combination	5 mg haloperidol + 25 mg promethazine (for individuals of small build/ lesser degree of disturbance)	IM	Repeated after half an hour	About 45–60 mg haloperidol/day
	10 mg haloperidol + 50 mg promethazine			
Zuclopenthixol acetate	50–150 mg	IM	Repeat after 24 hours after re-assessment of patient	Maximum of 400 mg over a 2-week period
Benzodiazepines				
Lorazepam	2–4 mg	Oral	Every 4–6 hours	10 mg/day
	2–4 mg	IM	Every 1–2 hours	10 mg/day

of the situation, the severity of the violence, and the level of cooperation of the patient.

Sedative medication is preferred when patients are agitated and disturbed. Oral medication can be employed for milder disturbance, while the parenteral route is preferred in severe violence. The newer antipsychotics are preferred as they have fewer extra-pyramidal adverse effects. Each country and center has its own regimen for sedation and control of violence and disturbed behavior. Studies for India and Brazil have shown that a combination of haloperidol and promethazine/midazolam can be effectively combined (in the same syringe) and produce a greater degree of sedation than other medication. Its advantages include its low cost. Other drugs that are employed include olanzapine, zuclopenthixol, etc. The newer antipsychotics are said to act faster, have fewer adverse effects, and result in less sedation and more calming of people who are disturbed. The newer medication is also available as mouth dissolving tablets or wafers. Lorazepam is the preferred benzodiazepine as it is reliably absorbed after intramuscular injection. Oral lorazepam is used as an adjunct to antipsychotic medication for sedation for patients with psychosis. It is also to be given for alcohol withdrawal and violence secondary to seizures.

While parenteral medication is given to non-cooperative patients, it is always preferable to persuade patients to cooperate. Forced administration of medication is justified only when the patient is in danger of harming himself and others as he/she is deemed to be not mentally competent to decide about treatment. Although consent for treatment is implied by relatives when they bring patients to the hospital or when patients are brought by the police, legal procedures should be followed and written consent may be necessary. In such situations, it is mandatory that the details of behavior are meticulously recorded.

A show of force quietens down many individuals, but others may require physical restraint. Patients with complex histories and severe violence may require referral to psychiatrists for further management.

CONCLUSION

Although the setting, evaluation, and management strategies in general hospital facilities may not be ideal, a degree of competence can be achieved with rehearsal and practice. While this chapter is divided into sub-headings for the sake of convenience, in actual practice the many components will have to be delivered simultaneously.

17 Crisis Intervention

People who experience psychological or medical crises and overwhelming stress often consult their physician. Physicians can help resolve the crisis by providing reassurance and support, evaluating the nature of the problem, determining the patient's mental state, ensuring the safety of the people involved, assisting the patient in developing an action plan to overcome difficulties, and providing follow-up consultation.

INTRODUCTION

People who experience psychological or medical crises often consult their physician. A crisis is defined as any event perceived as overwhelming by the patient, and may trigger a crisis reaction consisting of psychological and physiological symptoms. Patients visit general practitioners (GPs) when they are disturbed or distressed, when they are in pain, or are worried about the implication of their symptoms. Bereavement, marital discord, domestic violence, inability to cope at work, and financial problems can also lead people to seek help. This chapter briefly discusses the management of people in such difficulties.

How often do general physicians see patients in crisis?

About 1 in 20 patients attending a general medical setting or family practice presents a crisis and requires help and support from their physician. Although this may not appear to form a significant part of the physician's daily routine, the amount of time, effort, and skills required to resolve such situations mandate the need for specific training in the area. Accurate assessment and appropriate intervention are essential to ensure the safety of the people involved, to assist the patient in coping effectively with the problem, and to empower the patient to confront future life events.

What is a crisis?

A crisis occurs when a person is confronted with a critical event or stressful situation that is perceived as overwhelming. The incident or circumstance results in great distress despite the use of traditional problem-solving and coping strategies. Very often, it is not the event itself that causes the crisis; rather, it is the appraisal of the event as serious, uncontrollable, and beyond the patient's resources for coping that triggers a crisis response. People who are unable to cope with such events often seek a physician's assistance. Table 17.1 gives examples of events that can trigger crises.

158

TABLE 17.1

Examples of Events that can Trigger Crises

1. *Life-transition Events:* Birth of child, marriage, change in job/career, retirement

2. *Natural or Man-made Disasters:* Earthquake, floods, fires, riots, war

3. *Health-related/Medical:* Newly diagnosed disease or an exacerbation of a current medical problem, such as HIV infection, infertility, myocardial infarction, and cancer; medical problems that result in partial or total disability, psychiatric syndromes which affect coping

4. *Situational:* Bereavement, loss of job, motor vehicle collision, divorce, major family conflicts, and rape

5. *Existential Conflicts:* Realization that one will never make a significant impact on one's profession, remorse that one has never married or had children, despair that one's life has been meaningless

---

WHAT IS THE PHYSICIAN'S ROLE IN CRISIS RESOLUTION?

Patients experiencing a crisis often rely on their physician for support and advice. The physician's role includes providing reassurance and support to the patient, assessing the situation, ensuring the safety of the people involved, and teaching the patient strategies that will assist him/her to cope more effectively with the current incident as well as manage future stressful events.

WHAT ARE THE PRINCIPLES OF CRISIS INTERVENTION?

Patients, their stress, and their situations are different. Nevertheless, there are several general steps that physicians can follow to respond effectively to a patient's crisis. Physicians can help resolve the crisis by providing reassurance and support, evaluating the nature of the problem, determining the patient's mental state, ensuring the safety of the people involved, assisting the patient in developing an action plan to overcome difficulties, and providing follow-up consultation. Medication or referral for psychiatric or psychological counseling may be necessary in a minority of patients with continuing problems.

WHAT ARE THE SPECIFIC STEPS IN DEFUSING CRISES?

The steps are listed in Table 17.2. These general principles need to be tailored to the individual patient, the specific stress, and the particular situation.

TABLE 17.2

Steps in Crisis Management

1. Develop a rapport and provide support
2. Evaluate the magnitude of the crisis
3. Ensure safety
4. Stabilize the emotional state
5. Provide ongoing support

Step 1. Develop a rapport and provide support

The first step in managing a patient experiencing a crisis is to reassure him/her that it is safe to discuss the stress and concerns; that the physician will be available to help him/her through the crisis. Acknowledging distress shows empathy and is useful in establishing a therapeutic relationship. Active listening and encouraging the patient to discuss the issues and circumstances are necessary. The validation of the patient's experience in terms of understanding the context and providing support and empathy without taking sides or passing judgments is mandatory.

Making the patient comfortably seated and encouraging relaxation through deep breathing techniques is useful. Verbal techniques (*see also* Chapter 24 on Communication Skills) include the use of open-ended questions and encouraging statements. Repeating the last three words in order that the patient continues the conversation and is able to ventilate his or her concerns is a useful strategy. Non-verbal methods include good eye contact, leaning forwards, and nodding to show interest and concern. Such support and rapport will allow for the development of a therapeutic relationship.

Step 2. Evaluate the magnitude of the crisis

The next step is to evaluate the severity of the crisis. The context, the stress, the reactions, the attempts at coping, the coping strategies employed, the supports, and the implications have to be assessed. It is important to understand the issues from the patient's perspective.

The assessment will have to take into account the person's general appearance, physical health, and mental state. The exclusion of psychosis (strange beliefs, hearing voices, and grossly abnormal behavior) and substance use (alcohol, cannabis, and benzodiazepines) is mandatory. People with severe depression with a high suicidal risk require specific management. The factors that predict suicidal risk (*see also* Chapter 10 on Attempted Suicide) include older age, male sex, substance use, physical disease, psychiatric syndrome, and poor social supports.

The risk of violence and homicide should also be carefully examined. The patients at risk of violence include those with a history of antisocial traits, violence, and substance use. Patients at such risk should be directly asked about plans for violence and suicide. This information should also be confirmed with relatives and informants.

Step 3. Ensure safety

The evaluation of the severity of the crisis and its implications on the safety of the patient, the family, and others involved is crucial. People who risk harming themselves or others through violence should be identified. Those at higher risk would require hospitalization or close monitoring by relatives. Access to instruments, which can cause harm to self and to others, should be restricted. People without social supports and living alone and at risk for violence and suicide should be admitted to hospital. People with a high suicidal risk may require psychiatric referral.

Patients at low risk for violence and suicide, with stable family situations, and good social supports can be managed at home but with regular and frequent review.

Step 4. Stabilize the emotional state

The next step involves stabilization of the patient's emotional state. Facilitating understanding of the big picture, eliciting emotions, and confronting maladaptive coping mechanisms is crucial.

The doctor should elicit the current strategies used for coping with the stressful situation. It is crucial to consider alternative coping strategies to replace inappropriate coping methods, such as denial, withdrawal, and substance use. Negative thoughts, pessimism, and negative worldviews that lead to catastrophic generalizations should be recognized. Possible alternative strategies that may suggest a constructive response to the events should be considered. Emphasis should be placed on the fact that while the patient may not be able to control the stressful events, he/she can control the response to the situation.

General coping strategies should be discussed. Yoga, meditation, deep breathing exercises, muscle relaxation, leisure activities, and physical exercise, which reduce stress and improve coping, should be recommended. These should be incorporated into the patient's daily routine.

The physician and the patient should explore other alternative perspectives and approaches to deal with the crisis. Obtaining additional information, gathering situational support (e.g. family, friends), and using positive and constructive thinking patterns (i.e. those that change the patient's view of the problem) should be considered. Specific "homework" assignments on collecting additional information, monitoring of thoughts and activities, and the identification of strengths and experimentation with new coping behaviors can empower the patient to take action rather than feel helpless. The focus should be on exploring solutions, improving coping, and restoring function (Box 17.1).

Specific medication is required if the patient satisfies criteria for psychiatric

---

BOX 17.1   CRITICISM OF SINGLE SESSION DEBRIEFING

The majority of people who experience trauma due to natural disasters, lose loved ones in tragedies, and become victims of violence will not need assistance from mental health professionals. While most people are upset, distressed, and bereaved, these are normal human reactions and the majority will recover. Only a minority will have persistent psychological difficulties and need professional help to get back to normal life and functioning.

There is evidence to suggest that single session debriefing for people who have faced natural or humanmade disasters and severe trauma is not only ineffective but may worsen the person's condition. Many emotions elicited during the interview, the numerous conflicts discussed, and the several expectations raised demand continued support. Single session counseling and debriefing often leaves the patient distressed and stranded, without any further support, while the counselor has moved on to other projects. The World Health Organization does not support such practice.

syndromes. The short-term use of benzodiazepines may be necessary for people who have marked sleep disturbance. Sedative antidepressant medication (e.g. dothiepin/dosulepin, mirtazapine) is useful in those with severe anxiety and depression (*see also* Chapter 23 on Basic Psychotropic Medication Management). People who are dependent on alcohol will require a detoxification program with benzodiazepines and vitamins (*see also* Chapter on Substance Use). Patients with symptoms of psychosis will require antipsychotic medication (*see also* Chapter 8 on Psychosis).

Patients with a high risk of violence, suicide, and homicide will require hospitalization. Those who refuse voluntary admission to psychiatric facilities may require compulsory admission. It is always better to overestimate the risk and be safe than to underestimate it and be sorry later.

The physician can stabilize distress, explore other options, and make the patient commit to a plan. The patient and the doctor should develop a specific plan of action to manage the issues. The plan should be detailed and the steps clear so that the patient and the family are aware of the strategy. There should be a commitment on the part of the patient and the family to follow through with the plan. The action plan should be a short list of realistic, concrete, and positive steps, to be implemented as soon as is possible with the aim of stabilizing the patient, increasing his/her control over the situation, and promoting independent functioning. The patient should be encouraged to give up dysfunctional patterns and switch to the more positive approaches identified.

Step 5. Provide ongoing support

The support offered during the initial sessions should be continued in order to check on the patient's mental state and to reinforce his/her positive efforts to resolve the crisis. Crises usually tend to highlight danger, but they also provide opportunities to improve coping and consequently, functioning. The follow-up can ensure that the patient has made lasting changes so that he/she will be able to cope with similar stressors in the future.

Physicians should periodically review the progress, reinforce therapeutic gains, and elaborate and fine-tune the existing plans with the aim of increasing the patient's resilience. They should highlight the gains, and focus on the positive outcomes, improved self-discipline, and competence.

Patients who are not coping well despite continued support will require professional psychological support and should be referred to the community services available.

CONCLUSION

Although rare, patients who present with a crisis demand an extraordinary amount of time and resources on the part of the physician. Crisis intervention can be mastered with a little training, provide an invaluable service, and be a source of satisfaction to the physician.

18 Grief and Bereavement

People consult physicians during periods of stress such as bereavement. Recognizing the clinical presentation and the stage of grief is necessary. Establishing a rapport, acknowledging distress, allowing ventilation, eliciting the patient's perspectives, providing support, excluding medical disease, educating the patient and family about the issues involved, prescribing medication, if necessary, discussing stress, and helping the patient cope are crucial.

INTRODUCTION

People in distress often consult GPs and family physicians. Grief and bereavement is one such situation as the stress of losing relatives and friends is very painful. Grief presents with a variety of emotions, including shock, anger, sadness, and guilt. While these symptoms can be overwhelming and frightening, and it may appear as if the sadness will never let up, these are all part of the normal emotional reaction to loss.

WHAT IS GRIEF?

Grief is a natural response to loss. While grief is usually related to the death of a loved one, any loss can cause such suffering, including the break-up of a relationship, loss of employment, serious illness, miscarriage, and stillbirth.

The intensity of the grief is related to the significance of the loss. However, even subtle losses can lead to grief and are dependent on the personality and context. Moving away from home, graduating from college, changing jobs, and retiring from a career are examples.

IS GRIEF UNIFORM OR IS THERE DIVERSITY?

Everyone grieves differently. Grieving is a very personal and individual process and experience. The process is dependent on many factors, including personality, coping style, context, social supports, life experiences, religious faith, and the nature of the loss.

The grieving process takes time and the duration is variable. Healing usually takes place gradually; it cannot be forced or hurried. Some people start to feel better in weeks or months. For others, the grieving process is often measured in years. There is a need to accept the diversity of grieving and to be aware that normal grief is usually defined by cultural standards rather than by universal criteria.

BOX 18.1   MYTHS AND FACTS ABOUT GRIEF

MYTH: "The pain will go away faster if you ignore it."
Fact: Trying to ignore your pain or keeping it from surfacing may complicate matters. It is necessary to face the loss and deal with grief for healing to occur.

MYTH: "It's important to be strong in the face of loss."
Fact: Feeling sad, frightened, or lonely are normal reactions to loss. Crying does not imply weakness. Putting on a brave front and not showing one's true feelings can hinder the process of recovery.

MYTH: "If you don't cry, it means you aren't sorry about the loss."
Fact: Crying is the usual and normal response to sadness. However, different people express their sadness in different ways and the failure to cry does not imply a lack of pain or loss.

MYTH: "Grief should last about a year."
Fact: There is no definite time frame for grieving and there are wide variations in recovery. However, a review with a physician may be necessary if personal and social functioning continues to be severely impaired after a few months.

WHAT ARE THE MISCONCEPTIONS RELATED TO GRIEF?

Grief and bereavement are often misunderstood. Box 18.1 documents some myths and facts. Exploring the person's beliefs about grief and loss is necessary for understanding the person's context and coping.

WHAT ARE THE COMMON SYMPTOMS OF GRIEF?

Shock, disbelief, sadness, anger, guilt, and fear are common. Physical symptoms of tiredness, fatigue, and aches and pains are also usual. The sadness can extend to crying, loneliness, hopelessness, helplessness, and a lack of confidence. Disturbed sleep is common. Abuse of alcohol and medication is also frequent. Occasional suicidal ideation may occur and this has to be taken seriously if it is persistent and associated with plans. Guilt, especially if the relationship was ambivalent, may be present. Anger at life, with the doctors who were involved in caring for the deceased person, and with God may be also present. Anxiety about the future and panic attacks may occur.

ARE THERE STAGES OF GRIEF?

Elisabeth Kübler-Ross described the stages of grief based on her work with patients facing terminal illness. These have since been generalized to cover other types of grief. The stages of grief are denial, anger, bargaining, depression, and acceptance. Others have suggested three stages: shock, depression and acceptance.

The initial stage of grief is characterized by shock and an unwillingness to accept the loss. Anger can be an emotion that is frequently present. People facing their own death may attempt to bargain with God not to let the loss occur in exchange of changes in behavior and lifestyle. Gradually this gives way to sadness and depression. The final

BOX 18.2   THE MEDICALIZATION OF GRIEF AND BEREAVEMENT

The earlier editions of the American Psychiatric Association's Diagnostic and Statistical Manual (DSM) criteria for major depressive disorder had a bereavement exclusion clause. This meant that people who were grieving for the loss of their loved ones could not receive the label major depression, even if they seemed to satisfy the diagnostic criteria based on the DSM symptom checklist. However, the fifth edition of the DSM removed this exclusion making the possibility that people with normal grief reactions receive the label.

Many scholars have criticized the removal of the bereavement exclusion criteria and have argued that normal grief has been medicalized. They argue that by focusing on the symptom checklist it removes the impact of context and deemphasizes traditional and cultural methods of adapting to the loss. They suggest that this increases the risks of over diagnosis and over treatment. It also expands the market for pharmaceutical companies.

Fortunately, GPs and family physicians view patients in their contexts and recognize the importance of social supports and cultural ways of coping.

phase is one of acceptance, when the person starts to reintegrate with life; he/she makes new relationships and a fresh start.

These stages are not rigid phases of grief, nor are they sequential. Frequently, they are overlapping, with no distinct boundaries. Some of the characteristics described may be completely absent in certain people. Grief and bereavement can have marked fluctuations in sadness and related symptoms and can be like a roller coaster (Box 18.2). With time, the frequency, intensity, and duration of distress decrease.

STEPS IN MANAGEMENT

The following steps are useful:
1. Recognize presentation, establish rapport, allow ventilation, and provide support
2. Acknowledge distress
3. Allow ventilation, elicit the patient's perspective, and provide support
4. Take a focused history; carry out physical examination and laboratory investigations
5. Educate the patient and the family about the issues
6. Prescribe medication, if necessary
7. Suggest seeking additional support and general psychological strategies
8. Discuss specific stress
9. Discuss compliance, participation, and responsibility
10. Give an appointment for regular review.

Step 1. Recognize presentation, establish rapport, allow ventilation, and provide support

Patients may present to physicians during periods of grief and bereavement. Many will present with medically unexplained symptoms, while a few will mention the loss and the associated psychological distress. Routinely asking people with medically unexplained symptoms about stress often results in the identification of such presentations. Establishing a rapport, allowing ventilation, and providing support are important steps in management.

Step 2. Acknowledge distress

Acknowledging distress and the magnitude of the loss conveys that the physician has understood the context, is empathetic, and will help. This is an important step in establishing a therapeutic relationship.

Step 3. Allow ventilation, elicit the patient's perspectives, and provide support

Allowing the patient to talk about the issues, the death, its cause, the funeral, its aftermath and impact, and its implications is useful in understanding the context and the grief. Sharing grief usually helps unburden the patient. Eliciting the details of the relationship will allow the physician to assess the magnitude of the emotional loss. Listening to the person's point of view rather than trying to find out its accuracy is the aim of ventilation. Listening with compassion, sitting in silence without the need to keep the conversation going, and offering support without minimizing the loss are useful techniques. The provision and offer of support in the future will go a long way in alleviating distress.

Step 4. Take a focused history; carry out physical examination and laboratory investigations

Periods of grief and bereavement make people neglect their health. The period is also stressful and can precipitate or worsen many physical illnesses, including diabetes and hypertension. People going through such stress are prone to infections because of changes in immunity. Taking a focused history and carrying out a general physical examination and routine laboratory investigations will help identify new diseases and document the state of established conditions. Discussing compliance with medication, and encouraging a healthy diet and exercise are helpful.

Step 5. Educate the patient and the family about the issues

Many people may not be aware of the normalcy of their response, the symptoms of grief, its facts and myths, and its stages, duration, and progression. The variation in normal response, the diversity of responses to bereavement, should be mentioned. The usual process of recovery can be discussed.

Step 6. Prescribe medication, if necessary

Most patients manage without any medication. Sudden, unexpected, and unnatural deaths may cause a lot of distress, with significant insomnia. Allowing people under stress to get a good night's sleep will help them cope with the issues of the day. Benzodiazepines can be prescribed for short periods of a few weeks. It is better to consider antidepressants for persistent insomnia and severe depression. Sedative medication is preferred (e.g. dotheipin/dosulepin, mirtazapine). People may also benefit from vitamins as many neglect their diet.

Step 7. Suggest seeking additional support and general psychological strategies

The single most important factor in healing from loss is having the support of other people. Sharing loss and grief makes the burden easier to carry. Connecting to other people helps healing. Turning to friends and family, and drawing support from faith and religion are useful. Facing and accepting feelings, and expressing one's feelings and loss in tangible ways are necessary.

Psychological strategies, yoga, meditation, physical exercise, hobbies, and leisure are helpful for recovery. Religious activities for people with religious beliefs are useful. Planning for anniversaries of the loss, other milestones, and triggers that may worsen the grief and rekindle intense feelings is a good strategy. Those with extreme distress may need professional counseling.

Step 8. Discuss specific stress and coping

Specific issues may require problem-solving approaches. Loneliness, the lack of companionship, financial problems, coping with home and work, and coping with children and the emotional burden of becoming a single parent are common issues, which may need some discussion, especially in subsequent sessions. Specific solutions to particular problems will have to be given to the patient. The physician's role is often to show the big picture and the possible options rather than suggesting particular solutions.

Step 9. Discuss compliance, participation, and responsibility

Gradually, and with each subsequent review, the patient's compliance with the various suggestions will have to be enquired into. The patient will slowly, and after a few months of bereavement, have to take the responsibility of getting on with life and starting afresh, which most people are able to.

Step 10. Give an appointment for regular review

The provision of regular and long-term support may be necessary. Even brief, yet regular sessions are helpful to people who find it difficult to cope alone with their grief and those who have faced sudden and unnatural death and loss.

WHAT ARE THE WARNING SIGNS THAT GRIEF IS BECOMING COMPLICATED?

Complicated grief is defined as grief which is very severe and which causes incapacitating symptoms of depression, including marked insomnia, weight loss, inability to function, poor personal care, and suicidal ideation. Grief with prominent symptoms of depression and incapacitation for more than six months is also considered abnormal. People with persistent thoughts about suicide, those who make plans, and have made attempts will require help. Such presentations may require antidepressant medication and psychotherapy. Occasionally, people in bereavement can develop psychotic symptoms, such as persistent hallucinations, strange beliefs, and grossly abnormal behavior, and may require antipsychotic medication.

WHEN SHOULD I REFER FOR SPECIALIST INTERVENTION?

Referral for psychotherapy and for psychiatric help is usually for those with complicated grief, severe depression, and psychosis. Suicidal and homicidal risk should be carefully evaluated. The physician should enquire about such ideas, plans, and attempts, which should be taken very seriously, and referral should be considered. Those not responding to basic psychotropic and psychological support should be referred.

CONCLUSION

Many people with grief are distressed and seek medical help for a variety of reasons. Managing such patients can be very rewarding.

Section V

Common Clinical Presentations Among Children

19 Nocturnal Enuresis

Children with nocturnal enuresis are frequently brought to family physicians. The exclusion of medical, urological, and neurological causes is mandatory. Management includes the identification and resolution of psychosocial stress, restriction of water and fluids in the evenings, waking the child to pass urine at night, and reinforcement for dry nights with rewards. Antidepressant medication in small doses is useful.

INTRODUCTION

Enuresis is the repeated voiding of urine during the day or night into bed or clothes. Usually the voiding is involuntary, but occasionally it may be intentional. A diagnosis of enuresis implies that it is frequent (e.g. twice a week for three months), causes significant distress, and interferes with social or academic functioning. The child should have reached the age of 5 years, the age at which continence is expected. In children with developmental delays, the child should have a mental age of at least 5 years. The incontinence should not be due to medication (e.g. diuretic or sedative) or due to a medical condition (e.g. diabetes, spina bifida, and seizures).

Nocturnal enuresis, the commonest type of enuresis, is defined as the involuntary passage of urine during sleep in the absence of any identified physical abnormality in children above 5 years of age. Voiding in nocturnal enuresis usually takes place during rapid eye movement (REM) sleep, and the child may recall it as a dream that involved the act of urinating. It is common among boys and its prevalence reduces exponentially with age; children with such problems often present to general physicians. This chapter discusses a simple approach to managing such patients in primary care.

WHAT IS THE PREVALENCE OF ENURESIS?

The prevalence of enuresis is age dependent. It ranges from 5% to 10% among 5-year-olds, 3%–5% of 10-year-olds, and 1% of individuals over 15 years age are said to have the condition. Enuresis can be classified into primary and secondary.

WHAT IS THE DEVELOPMENT AND COURSE OF ENURESIS?

Two types of enuresis have been described. Primary enuresis is when the child has not achieved any degree of control over bladder function, i.e. never established urinary continence. Secondary enuresis is diagnosed when bladder control is achieved for a few months or years, after which there is a loss of control.

The most common time for the onset of secondary incontinence is between 5 and

TABLE 19.1

Common Causes of Enuresis

1. *Urological Conditions*
   a. Urological abnormalities and obstruction, e.g. urethral valves, meatal stenosis, and bladder neck obstruction
   b. Recurrent urinary infections
2. *Neurological Problems*
   a. Spinal bifida
   b. Spinal tumors
   c. Epilepsy
   d. Mental retardation
3. *Medical Causes*
   a. Diabetes mellitus
   b. Diabetes insipidus
4. *Medication Effects* (e.g. diuretics, antipsychotic medication, sedatives)
5. *Psychological Stress as cause*
   a. Problems for the child, including sibling rivalry, academic difficulties
   b. Problems at home, including marital discord, single parent situations, inconsistent or very strict discipline, physical, emotional, and sexual abuse

8 years of age, but it can occur at any age. However, most children with the disorder are continent by adolescence.

The causes of primary and daytime enuresis after the age of 5 years are mainly medical, neurological, and urological, while those of secondary loss of bladder control are often psychogenic. This distinction can be made after eliciting a brief history.

WHAT ARE THE CAUSES OF ENURESIS?

There are many causes for enuresis and these are listed in Table 19.1. The child will have to be examined to rule out common medical and neurological causes.

WHAT INVESTIGATIONS ARE NECESSARY TO RULE OUT MEDICAL CAUSES?

Primary and daytime incontinence after the age of 5 years suggests the possibility of a physical disease, while nocturnal and secondary enuresis suggests psychological causation and implies environmental stress. Consequently, primary and daytime enuresis will require appropriate neurological and urological investigations. Recurrent urinary tract infection (UTI) can be ruled out using urine microscopy. The identification of specific causes for the lack of bladder control mandates specific treatment for the identified cause.

WHAT ARE THE PSYCHOLOGICAL CAUSES OF ENURESIS?

The majority of children who present to primary care have secondary enuresis. A variety of psychological stressors are associated with enuresis. The birth of a sibling, sibling rivalry, and academic difficulties are commonly reported in children with enuresis. Problems at home, which can cause stress and enuresis, include marital discord, single parent situations, inconsistent or very strict discipline, and physical, emotional, and sexual abuse.

WHAT ARE THE STEPS IN MANAGEMENT?

The ten steps in management are:

1. Recognize the clinical presentation
2. Acknowledge distress
3. Elicit the patient's and the family's perspective
4. Carry out physical examination and laboratory investigations to rule out medical problems
5. Educate the family about the nature of illness and its treatment
6. Prescribe medication
7. Discuss the role of stress as cause and consequence of illness
8. Elaborate coping strategies
9. Negotiate a treatment plan, compliance, participation, and responsibility
10. Give an appointment for review.

Step 1. Recognize the clinical presentation and elicit clinical details

The nature and frequency of the enuresis in relation to age has to be elicited from the parents. Specifically, elicit the details of whether there were periods when partial or complete bladder control was achieved and the circumstances of the loss of control. Details of sleep arrangements and parental attitudes to the enuresis should be elicited.

The possibility of stress, including marital discord, single parent situations, academic stress, issues related to inconsistent and very strict discipline, physical, and sexual abuse, and sibling rivalry, needs to be explored. Primary enuresis (with complete absence of bladder control without any significant period during which the child has been dry) should be differentiated from secondary enuresis (where control was achieved and the child was dry for at least six months). Similarly, enuresis during sleep should be distinguished from incontinence during periods when the child is awake.

Step 2. Acknowledge distress

Enuresis is distressing both for children and the parents. Acknowledging distress, while offering support and treatment, is helpful in management.

Step 3. Elicit the child's and the family's perspective

The child and the family will have opinions on the cause of the problem. Eliciting these perspectives will give the physician insights into the psychological environment at home. While parents can be directly asked about any stress that the child is facing and any problems at home, such direct questioning may not work with children. The "three wishes test" is a useful tool for bringing out conflicts plaguing a child. It may be useful to put such wishes in the context of religion, as most families are religious. For example, "If you prayed/went to the temple and God granted you three wishes, what would you choose?"; very often the child will mention the areas of conflict and stress in the list of wishes.

Step 4. Physical examination and laboratory investigations

Urological conditions (e.g. urological abnormalities and obstruction such as urethral valves, meatal stenosis, bladder neck obstruction, and recurrent urinary infections), medical conditions (e.g. diabetes mellitus and insipidus), and neurological problems (e.g. spinal bifida, spinal tumors, epilepsy and mental retardation) are common causes for the inability to achieve bladder control in childhood; these have to be excluded. The possibility of a UTI can be ruled out with a simple test for urine microscopy. Details of medications used are necessary to exclude medication related effects (e.g. diuretics, antipsychotics, and sedatives). The identification of specific causes for the lack of bladder control mandates specific treatment for the identified cause. Primary and daytime incontinence after the age of 5 years suggests the possibility of a physical disease, while secondary and nocturnal enuresis suggests psychological causation and implies environmental stress.

Step 5. Educate the patient about the nature of illness and treatment

Educating the child and family about the nature of the problem is crucial. Primary enuresis with medical causes should be explained. Recurrent UTI would necessitate appropriate antibiotic therapy. Urological and neurological causes will require specific referral to specialists for appropriate interventions.

Psychological causation, the impact of stress, and enuresis as a maladaptive coping mechanism need to be highlighted. One should emphasize the need for the resolution of conflicts and the reduction of the stress to bring about an improvement.

Step 6. Prescribe medication

Placebos (e.g. vitamin tablets and syrups) are sometimes used along with other measures, such as positive reinforcement, the reduction of stress, and the resolution of conflict. However, placebos are short-term solutions, and the resolution of conflicts and stress is required for long-term success.

Tricyclic antidepressants (e.g. imipramine and amitriptyline) are useful for children with long-standing nocturnal enuresis. Small doses of 12.5–25 mg at bedtime for a period of 3–6 months help many children. This should be used in combination with other measures.

Step 7. Discuss the role of stress in causation

Psychological stress is commonly associated with nocturnal enuresis. Exploring stress at home and at school is a vital part of management. The identification of the sources of anxiety, including marital discord, single parent situations, academic stress, issues related to inconsistent and very strict discipline, physical and sexual abuse, and sibling rivalry, and their resolution is mandatory. Parents should be advised on problem solving and the need for reduction of conflicts at home and at school for improvement in the child's nocturnal enuresis. Often enuresis is the child's attempt at resolving stress, which he/she cannot handle. Discussing the connection between nocturnal enuresis and stress, and encouraging the parents to address these issues are cardinal to success.

Step 8. Elaborate coping strategies

The first step is to maintain a detailed record of baseline nocturnal enuresis to assess the progress. The parents or relatives should be encouraged to maintain a diary of events and their relationship to nocturnal enuresis.

The parents should be advised to restrict the fluid intake of the child in the evening and before bedtime. Voiding before sleep is essential to prevent nocturnal enuresis. Similarly, interrupting sleep by waking up the child to allow him/her to void is helpful. The child should be completely awake before he/she passes urine so that he/she is aware of the process.

The parents should be encouraged to maintain a star chart or calendar. Dry nights should be marked with red stars, while those with the incontinence, without. Lavish praise on the child for dry nights and tell him or her that obtaining stars is important. A material reward (e.g. chocolates, ice cream, and books) for dry periods of 3–5 days will go a long way in reinforcing such behavior. Punishment and shaming usually make the problem worse and should be avoided.

The reduction of stress and the resolution of conflicts at home are mandatory for success. Issues related to the consistency of discipline rather than its harsh implementation should be discussed. Sibling rivalry should be addressed. Strategies, which employ praise and giving increased attention to the child for periods of good behavior, while ignoring bad behavior, are useful. The reduction of academic pressures and expectations at school and at home may be necessary for children who are not coping well with their studies. Some may require additional help and support to cope with the huge burden of studies, which is common in India.

The resolution of marital discord and conflict at home is necessary. Other stressors should be explored and examined, and strategies for their resolution considered.

Step 9. Negotiate a treatment plan, compliance, participation, and responsibility

The treatment plan should be negotiated with the child and the parents. The new dietary and voiding schedules, the star chart, and reinforcement schedules should be discussed with the child. Encouraging the child to take responsibility for his/her bladder control is necessary.

Discussing the responsibility of parents and guardians in exploring, identifying and reducing stress, and resolving conflicts through healthy strategies is mandatory for success. Reiterating the connection between nocturnal enuresis and stress is necessary. Parents should be encouraged to solve these problems and resolve conflicts.

Step 10. Give an appointment for review

The appointment for review is to monitor progress. The child should be praised for even small progress and should be encouraged to take control of his/her bladder. The measures to prevent enuresis and the positive reinforcement strategies should be reviewed. The reduction of stress and the resolution of conflicts should be discussed with the parents. Medication can be prescribed, if necessary.

BOX 19.1   ENURESIS

Mr and Ms X visited their family physician along with their two children. They complained that their older boy, aged 5 years, had recently started wetting his bed at night. He had attained good bladder control for over six months but lost it after his younger sister was born two months ago. They also mentioned that he is jealous of his sister and had occasionally hurt her. Since her birth, they had been busy looking after their little daughter and had been spending less time with their son.

The parents were helped to understand the child's situation – the change from being the center of all attention to losing center-stage to his little sister. It was suggested that they spend equal time with the boy and encourage him to talk about the new situation in the family. The amount of fluids drunk in the evenings was controlled and the boy was encouraged to pass urine before going to bed and he was woken up from his sleep to pass urine. A star chart and rewards for dry nights helped him to regain bladder control.

WHEN SHOULD THE CHILD BE REFERRED FOR SPECIALIST HELP?

Primary enuresis may require specialist assessment and intervention. Secondary nocturnal enuresis that does not respond to the treatment mentioned should be referred to a specialist.

CONCLUSION

Enuresis is a common presentation in children. It is essential to identify that which is due to physical causes and that which is secondary to psychological problems. Simple strategies for management include alteration in some habits, dealing with stress, and prescribing medication, if necessary. Helping parents manage children with enuresis can be rewarding for physicians.

20 Temper Tantrums and Behavioral Problems

Children with behavioral problems are brought to family physicians for help and treatment. There is a need to understand the family context, the nature of the behavioral problems, and the precipitating and perpetuating factors. Issues related to discipline, strictness, consistency, punishment, reinforcement, and rewards should be elicited.

Developmental delay, hyperactivity, chronic physical illness, and hearing and vision problems will need to be diagnosed and managed. Managing tantrums and reinforcement of good behavior are discussed.

INTRODUCTION

Temper tantrums describe a range of behaviors in children, which are difficult to manage. The behavior can involve shouting, screaming, hitting, kicking, rolling on the floor, and even holding one's breath. Parents often seek help from physicians, as children are difficult to manage during these episodes. Temper tantrums are equally common in boys and girls, and usually occur between the ages of 1 and 5 years.

These outbursts are typically in response to frustration and can be verbal or behavioral (e.g. aggression). These may be isolated events or occur as a pattern of behavior seen consistently over time and in a variety of settings. Such behavior is developmental age inappropriate. Other conditions, such as intellectual disability, autism, and attention deficit hyperactivity disorders (ADHD) need to be excluded.

HOW COMMON ARE TEMPER TANTRUMS?

Occasional tempter tantrums are seen in many children, but the majority soon learn to handle their frustration. Severe and frequent disruptive behavior is much less common. Some reports mention a prevalence of 2%–5% range and are said to be more common in boys and in schoolgoing children than in girls and adolescents.

WHAT IS THE CAUSE FOR TEMPER TANTRUMS?

Occasional tantrums are a normal part of childhood. However, regular and severe tantrums suggest that the child is frustrated by his/her inability to get his/her own way. These imply that he/she is not able to handle the situation when his/her desires are not fulfilled. It means that the child is not able to communicate effectively and is unable to negotiate the issue involved.

The ten steps in management are:

1. Recognize the clinical presentation
2. Acknowledge distress
3. Elicit the patient's and the family's perspective
4. Take a focused history; carry out physical examination and laboratory investigations
5. Educate the family about the nature of illness and its treatment
6. Prescribe medication
7. Discuss the role of stress as cause and consequence of illness
8. Elaborate coping strategies
9. Negotiate a treatment plan, compliance, participation, and responsibility
10. Give an appointment for review.

Step 1. Recognize the clinical presentation and elicit details

One must ask the parents about the nature, severity, and frequency of the tantrums. The triggers, which start the process, the factors, which terminate it, and the consequences of such behavior need to be identified. The impact of temper tantrums on the child, his/her family, friends, and peers should be recognized.

Step 2. Acknowledge distress

Temper tantrums that are severe and occur often are distressing for parents. Tantrums often occur in public places and can be very embarrassing. Repeated tantrums at home disrupt the family, and are demoralizing for parents who do not know how to manage the child and the disruptive behavior. Acknowledging the distress caused, and offering support and treatment are essential.

Step 3. Elicit the child's and the parents' perspective

The child and the parents will have opinions on the cause of the problem. Eliciting these perspectives will give the physician insights into the psychological environment at home. Issues related to discipline, strictness, consistency, punishment, reinforcement, and rewards should be elicited.

While the parents can be directly asked about any stress that the child is facing and any problems at home, such direct questioning may not work with children. The "three wishes test" is a useful tool for bringing out conflicts troubling a child. It may be useful to put such wishes in the context of religion as most families are religious; for example, "If you prayed/went to the temple and God granted you three wishes, what would you choose?"; very often the child will mention the areas of conflict and stress.

Step 4. Take a focused history; carry out physical examination and laboratory investigations

A detailed history which analyses the behavior including antecedents, circumstances, situations, precipitants, and consequences, is mandatory. Developmental delays in children suggest intellectual disability and disorders such as autism (abnormal behavior, and poor socialization). Problems in vision and hearing and chronic physical illness can also contribute to tantrums. Inability to concentrate on tasks and marked restlessness may be suggestive of hyperactivity. While these conditions can also be treated with this protocol, which essentially focuses on the problem behavior, the child may also require specialist help to manage the underlying conditions.

Step 5. Educate the patient about the nature of illness and treatment

It is crucial to educate the child and family about the nature of the problem. Psychological causation and the fact that temper tantrums are maladaptive patterns of coping need to be highlighted. The need for consistency of discipline and a planned and unified strategy to manage discipline between parents is mandatory for improvement; this needs to be emphasized. The analysis of the situations, triggers, and consequences should be fed back to the parents, highlighting inconsistencies in approaches to disciplining the child.

Step 6. Prescribe medication

No medication is necessary for temper tantrums in normal children. Using placebos (e.g. vitamin tablets and syrups) along with common sense measures, positive reinforcement of appropriate behavior, and consistency of discipline go a long way in reducing the problem. However, placebos are short-term solutions and the proper handling of behavior and of discipline is required for long-term success.

Children with mental retardation, seizures, psychosis, autism, and hyperactivity may benefit from appropriate treatment for the control of the underlying problems. The control of seizures would necessitate anticonvulsant medication, while autism, psychosis, and hyperactivity may require small doses of antipsychotic medication (tab. haloperidol 0.25 mg twice a day; tab. risperidone 0.5 mg at bedtime). These conditions may require specialist treatment and referral.

Step 7. Discuss the role of stress as cause and consequence of behavior

Psychological stress may be associated with inconsistent and very strict discipline; physical abuse may be temporally related to the behavior problem. Parents should be advised on problem solving and the need for consistent discipline to produce an improvement in the child's behavior. Often the behavioral problem is the child's attempt at resolving his/her inability to handle frustration, poor communication, and negotiation. Discussing the connection between the problem behavior and the management of the issues related to discipline, reinforcement, and rewards is cardinal to success.

Step 8. Elaborate coping strategies

The maintenance of a detailed record of baseline temper tantrums is helpful in assessing progress. The parents or relatives should be encouraged to maintain a diary of events and their relationship to the tantrums.

Simple common sense measures for prevention should be discussed. Simple strategies, usually helpful in avoiding tantrums, should be elaborated. Providing enough attention to the child so that he/she does not seek attention through the tantrum is important. Giving the child a choice in making small decisions so that he/she feels a sense of control. Not providing any choices will only increase the child's frustration. Objects that can hurt the child should be kept out of sight. Distracting the child, when a tantrum is imminent, is a useful strategy. Providing opportunities for the child to achieve a sense of mastery by giving age-appropriate toys and games is useful. Recognizing fatigue, hunger, and the need for sleep and taking appropriate action can prevent tantrums. Some tantrums are not worth fighting against, but if the behavior puts the child or others at risk (e.g. biting and throwing items) then one should definitely intervene. Patents should be consistent with discipline and choose their battles carefully.

Positive reinforcement is a useful strategy to control behavior. The parents should be encouraged to maintain a star chart or calendar. Days without tantrums should be marked with red stars and those with tantrums without stars. Lavishing praise for good behavior and providing stars are mandatory. A material reward (e.g. chocolates, ice cream and books) for good behavior of 3–5 days will help in reinforcing such behavior. Punishment and shaming usually make the problem worse.

Advice on managing tantrums is essential. Parents and relatives should be reassured that temper tantrums are common in children and can be managed with simple measures. It is important to keep calm as getting upset, frustrated, or using physical punishment only complicates matters and worsens an already difficult situation. Trying to see the issues from the child's point to view to understand the

---

BOX 20.1   TEMPER TANTRUMS DUE TO FRUSTRATION

Ms A visited her doctor with her 18-month-old son. She described episodes where he threw terrible tantrums. For example, when he did not want to do something, he often threw himself on the floor, and kicked his arms and legs. She admitted that she could barely bring herself to take him out in public because he threw tantrums so often.

Ms A was helped to understand why her toddler threw tantrums. It was explained to her that a toddler has an intense desire to do things, but his mental and motor skills have developed more quickly than his ability to communicate. Because he did not yet have the verbal skills to express his frustration, he did so by throwing tantrums.

She was encouraged to stay calm, show empathy, reassure the child, and spend time to bond. The child was encouraged to communicate his feelings and desires using words and body language. The mother was encouraged to spend more time with the boy when he behaved well and reinforce such behavior with praise and rewards, while reducing attention during periods of bad behavior.

situation and the cause of the frustration is helpful in managing the tantrum. Providing comfort prophylactically and calming the child in the face of disappointment can prevent disruptive behavior. Ensuring that the child's environment is safe allows for ignoring some tantrums. Taking the child to a calm place for him/her to cool down is important. Discussing viable options and planning strategies to overcome obstacles

BOX 20.2 TEMPER TANTRUMS USED TO MANIPULATE PARENTS

Ms B visited her doctor with her son who was a clever and lovable 3-year-old. She mentioned that her son regularly threw tantrums. He regularly had episodes during which he cried, screamed, stiffened his limbs, arched his back, kicked, fell down, flailed about, or ran away. He also occasionally held his breath and broke things as part of a tantrum. These tantrums were precipitated when his desires were denied. She said that they stopped as soon as his wishes were satisfied. She had been giving in to all his wishes, even unreasonable ones, as she could not stand the disturbance.

The importance of staying calm, waiting the tantrum out, and making sure that it did not pay was explained to the mother; it was pointed out that giving in halfway through a tantrum sends a wrong message and greater disturbance will succeed. She was advised to reward positive behavior and encourage the child to express himself. She was reassured that soon the child would learn that tantrums do not pay, and the tantrums would decrease in frequency.

BOX 20.3 SIMPLE STRATEGIES TO AVOID TEMPER TANTRUMS

- Make sure that the child is getting enough attention so that he/she does not seek attention through the tantrum.
- Give the child a choice in making small decisions so that he/she feels a sense of control (e.g. "Do you want apple juice or mango juice?"), rather than no choice at all.
- Keep those objects, which the child should not play with, out of sight.
- Distract the child when it appears that he/she is going to start throwing a tantrum.
- Provide age-appropriate toys and games so that the child achieves a sense of mastery.
- Parents should recognize when the child is tired, hungry, or sleepy and take appropriate action.
- Parents should choose their battles carefully. Some tantrums are not worth fighting against while, on the other hand, if the behavior puts the child or others at risk (e.g. biting and throwing items), then one should definitely intervene. Parents should be consistent with discipline.

with gentle reasoning may also help. It is cardinal that children are not rewarded for the bad behavior, as this will only reinforce the association between such tantrums and returns. Offering praise for his/her calming down is useful.

Step 9. Negotiate a treatment plan, compliance, participation, and responsibility

The treatment plan should be negotiated with the child and the parents. The star chart and reinforcement schedules should be discussed with the child. Encouraging the child to take responsibility for his/her behavior is necessary.

Discussing the responsibility of parents and guardians in exploring, identifying, and reducing inconsistencies in enforcing discipline is mandatory for success. It is also necessary for the adults in the house to resolve their conflicts. Reiterating the connection between behavior problems and the family environment is useful. Parents should be encouraged to resolve these differences in opinions and child rearing practices. Resolving other conflicts and providing a consistent environment at home is crucial.

BOX 20.4   ADVICE TO MANAGE TANTRUMS

- Keep calm. Getting upset, frustrated, or using physical punishment only complicates matters.
- Try to understand the situation and the cause of the tantrum.
- Calm the child and help him/her face the disappointment; provide comfort.
- Ignoring some tantrums helps, but always be around to ensure that the child is safe.
- Gentle reasoning and giving viable options may also help.
- Take the child to a calm place to cool down.
- Offer praise for the child calming down after a tantrum.
- Do not reward tantrums.

BOX 20.5   THE MEDICALIZATION OF TEMPER TANTRUMS

The American Psychiatric Association's Diagnostic and Statistical Manual 5 (2013) includes a new category of Disruptive Mood Dysregulation Disorder (DMDD) for children with severe and frequent temper tantrums. The arguments for the usefulness of the label include the need to manage disruptive children in schools, and by the legal system. Many of these children currently seem to receive the label of bipolar disorder, which most psychiatrists agree is inappropriate. Its high prevalence was employed to justify the need for recognition. However, many critics have argued that it is based on limited research evidence and that the label medicalizes temper tantrums. It will also encourage the use of psychotropic medication and play into the hands of the pharmaceutical industry.

Step 10. Give an appointment for review

The appointment for review is to monitor progress. The child should be praised for even small progress and should be encouraged to take control of his/her emotions. The measures to prevent tantrums and the positive reinforcement strategies should be reviewed.

WHEN SHOULD CHILDREN BE REFERRED?

Children, who are in danger of hurting themselves, are destructive, and in whose case the above strategies do not work require specialist help. Specialist help may be necessary for managing intellectual disability, epilepsy, psychosis, autism, and hyperactivity disorders.

CONCLUSION

Simple details lie between success and failure. Teaching parents about the need for consistent discipline and helping them manage children with temper tantrums can be rewarding for physicians.

21 Learning Disability in Children

Children with normal intelligence can have problems in school related to learning due to specific learning disability. The problems can be related to reading, writing, math, fine motor skills, and auditory and visual processing. Intellectual disability, hyperactivity, and autism have to be excluded. The child will need special assessment and management by the school counselor or educational psychologist.

INTRODUCTION

Schooling and educational systems are stressful for many children. Some children find it difficult to cope with the standards demanded by the system and the rising expectations of parents. Consequently, the failure to meet the expected standards in school results in stress, ridicule for the child, and anxiety, and pressure for concerned parents. There are many causes for below-average performance of children in school. This chapter focuses on learning disability and related issues.

WHAT IS LEARNING DISABILITY?

Parents and many teachers mention the lack of attention in class, the reduced motivation to learn, the absence of focus, and deficit in hard work as characteristics of children with learning disability. A child with a learning disability, or learning disorder, does not have a problem with his/her general intelligence. Learning disorders are caused by differences in the brain that affect how information is received, processed, or communicated. The organization of the brain of children with such problems is different; it changes at a different pace, requires different input for growth, and is capable of much learning.

SYMPTOMS AND TYPES OF LEARNING DISABILITIES

There are different types of learning difficulties:

1. *Dyslexia:* The child has difficulty in processing language. The resultant problems include difficulties in reading, writing, spelling, and speaking. Basic reading problems occur when there is difficulty understanding the relationship between sounds, letters, and words. Reading comprehension problems occur when there is an inability to grasp the meaning of words, phrases, and paragraphs. Signs of reading difficulty include problems with letter and word recognition,

understanding words and ideas, reading speed and fluency, and difficulties with general vocabulary skills.

The child may read single words aloud incorrectly, slowly, and with hesitation. Reading requires a lot of effort and the child may frequently guess difficult sounding words. Some children while reading correctly may have difficulty in understanding the meaning of the text, its sequence, relationships, inferences, and subtleties. Some children have difficulties with spelling and may add, omit, or substitute vowels or consonants. The difficulty may be mild, moderate, or severe.

2. *Dyscalculia:* The predominant difficulty is with math. The child has trouble with mathematical problems, in understanding time, and in using money. A child with a math-based learning disorder may struggle with memorization and organization of numbers, operation signs, and number "facts" (such as 3+3=6 or 3×3=9). Children with math learning disorders might also have trouble with counting principles (such as counting by 2s or counting by 5s) or have difficulty telling time. The child may tend to count his/her fingers and get lost in computation.

The difficulty with math reflects issues in mathematical reasoning. The child may struggle to apply mathematical concepts, facts and procedures, and consequent difficulty in solving quantitative problems. Child can exhibit a variety of problems, which may lie on a spectrum of difficulty with mild, moderate, and severe disability and dysfunction.

3. *Dysgraphia:* The child has difficulty with writing. The problems with handwriting and spelling, and with organizing ideas, are obvious. They include problems with neatness and consistency of writing and spelling, with the accuracy of copying letters and words, and difficulties in the organization of writing and coherence. Written expression may lack clarity due to errors in grammar and punctuation. The organization of paragraphs may be poor.

4. *Dyspraxia:* This implies difficulty with fine motor skills and the integration of sensory stimuli due to problems with hand–eye coordination, balance, and manual dexterity. The child has problems with movement and coordination, whether it is with fine motor skills (cutting, writing) or gross motor skills (running, jumping).

5. *Auditory Processing Disorder:* The child has difficulty hearing the differences between sounds and this results in problems in reading, comprehension, and language. The inability to distinguish subtle differences in sound, or hearing sounds at the wrong speed, makes it difficult to sound out words and understand the basic concepts of reading, writing, and spelling.

6. *Visual Processing Disorder:* The child has problems in interpreting visual information, which results in difficulties with reading and math, recognizing symbols and pictures, and in interpreting charts and maps. Problems in visual perception include missing subtle differences in shapes, reversing letters or numbers, skipping words, skipping lines, misperceiving depth or distance, or having problems with eye–hand coordination.

These difficulties affect the child's academic skills, which are substantially below the expected range for his/her chronological age. It may not only cause problems in scholastic performance but also the child's activities of daily living. The difficulty begins in school age but may become more obvious with increased academic load, timed tests, and submission deadlines. These difficulties should be persistent and not transitory.

These problems should not be accounted for as intellectual disability, vision, or hearing difficulty, mental or neurological disorders, and psychosocial adversity.

RELATED PROBLEMS AND ISSUES

Children with learning difficulties also face other problems as a consequence of their learning problems. These children may have trouble expressing their feelings, calming themselves down, and reading non-verbal cues, which can lead to difficulty in the classroom and with their peers. They lack the social and emotional skills necessary to get along with other students and succeed in school. Academic challenges may lead to low self-esteem, withdrawal, and behavioral problems. Such difficulties need to be countered by creating a strong support system for such children and helping them learn to express themselves, deal with frustration, and work through challenges. The teachers and parents should focus on the growth of the child as a person, and not just on his/her academic achievements. This will help the child learn good emotional habits and the right tools for lifelong success.

OTHER DISORDERS THAT MAKE LEARNING DIFFICULT

Difficulty in school does not always stem from a learning disability. Anxiety, depression, stressful events, emotional trauma, and other conditions affecting concentration make learning a challenge. In addition, some other diseases have to be excluded:

1. *Attention-deficit Hyperactivity Disorder (ADHD):* ADHD, while not considered a learning disability, can certainly disrupt learning. Children with ADHD often have problems with sitting still, staying focused, following instructions, staying organized, and completing homework. They are restless and fidgety, have short attention spans, and are often disruptive in class.
2. *Autism:* Children with an autism spectrum disorder may have trouble making friends, reading body language, communicating, and making eye contact. These conditions affect many aspects of development, are pervasive, and include autism and Asperger syndrome.
3. *Intellectual Disability:* Children with problems with general intelligence will also present with difficulties in coping with early schooling. They will also have delays in developmental milestones: motor, speech, communication, self-help skills, socialization, etc. They are usually unable to cope with regular school and drop out. Children with gross and global intelligence problems, and deficits (i.e. intelligence quotient <70) will require individual and special input and training.

CAN GIFTED CHILDREN HAVE A LEARNING DISORDER?

Many characteristics of gifted children, both social and emotional, are mistaken as symptoms of specific learning disorders. Consequently, many gifted and talented children are often misdiagnosed as having learning disabilities or behavior disorders.

In addition, children with high IQ (e.g. >140), can have major differences between their verbal and performance intelligence, and can possess characteristics of learning disability. Often these children have unusual learning styles, and even though they are very intelligent, they may have learning disorders. They will benefit from extra support, encouragement, and intervention.

DIAGNOSIS OF LEARNING DISABILITY

The diagnosis of specific learning disability is complex and requires a detailed assessment. The child should be referred to the school counselor, a clinical psychologist, or a child psychiatrist for evaluation.

WHAT IS THE PREVALENCE OF LEARNING DISABILITY?

The prevalence of specific learning disability across the domains of reading, writing, and mathematics ranges between 5% and 15% of schoolgoing children. Its prevalence in adults is about 4%. Learning disability is more common among boys than among girls.

WHAT IS THE COURSE OF LEARNING DISORDERS?

While the ability of children with specific learning disorders may improve with age, problems with reading fluency, comprehension, spelling, written expression, and numeracy skills may persist into adulthood. The manifestation of the disability may change over time.

ARE THERE CULTURAL DIFFERENCES?

Specific learning disorders vary across languages, cultures, and socioeconomic classes. In languages such as Spanish and German, where there is a direct mapping of sounds and letters and non-alphabetic languages such as Chinese and Japanese, the hallmark of learning disability is slow but accurate reading. The linguistic and cultural context should be taken into account during assessment.

SUGGESTIONS FOR PARENTS

The following suggestions will help parents of children with learning disabilities:

- Emphasize good lifestyle habits, including healthy food, adequate sleep, and regular exercise.
- Support the child and help him/her to identify and manage anger, frustrations, and failure.
- Take charge of your child's education by identifying the specific problem and helping him/her learn solutions, and pursue a home program.
- Recognize the limitations of the school systems and work with the teachers.
- Identify your child's learning strengths and weaknesses. Focus on the strengths.
- Take a long-term view and emphasize success in life rather than at school.
- Be proactive and encourage self-awareness, esteem, and confidence.
- Set reasonable goals and persevere.

BOX 21.1 DYSLEXIA

Ms A, the mother of a bright and charming eight-year-old boy, reported that he was doing badly at school. Reading and writing were particularly difficult. He was clever with his hands but homework was a problem. His teacher mentioned that his spelling was poor and he frequently interchanged "p" for "q" and "d" for "b". He tended to omit short words and frequently guessed words, making errors. The mother had spoken to his teacher, who felt that her son was not working hard in class.

BOX 21.2 CRITIQUE OF THE MEDICAL MODEL OF LEARNING DISABILITY

Learning disability theory is based on the medical model which attributes such difficulty to biological causes in the brain. However, scholars examining the social, cultural, and structural causes argue otherwise. They suggest that the premium placed on literacy and numeracy in capitalistic societies is based on the economic system's need for efficiency and its emphasis on science. On the other hand, agrarian economies do not place such importance on reading, writing, and math as essential measure of adult adequacy. The fact that the rates of these disorders are much higher among minority groups argues that the diversity in cultural background of children is not taken into consideration. Similarly, the higher rates among children from lower socioeconomic strata of society supports structural causes of disability and disadvantage.

Many children with learning disabilities are able to compensate for their deficits and lead productive lives. Countries with progressive education policies allow for inclusive education of children with specific learning disability in their regular schools. They also provide additional teaching support, different curricula, and examination systems. However, such progressive learning environment varies across countries, regions, socioeconomic context, cultures, and medium of instruction. Such children should be encouraged to stay in regular schools, take up courses which suit them, and obtain equivalent qualifications.

22 Other Clinical Presentations in Childhood

Children with intellectual disability, autism, attention-deficit/hyperactivity, and stuttering are brought to general practitioners and family physicians. The recognition of these clinical syndromes, education about the nature of the illness, and support are helpful. Referral to specialist is required for detailed assessment and care.

INTRODUCTION

There are other clinical presentations in childhood that come to the attention of GPs and family physicians. These problems can cause significant distress to the child, their families, friends, and peers. These affect academic performance and activities of daily living. The clinical presentations, which need to be recognized, are briefly highlighted. These will require referral for detailed assessment and management. The clinical presentations include: (i) intellectual disability; (ii) autism spectrum; (iii) attention deficit/hyperactivity; and (iv) stuttering.

INTELLECTUAL DISABILITY

The child has deficits in intellectual functioning, which result in impairment in general mental abilities and adaptive functions in comparison to age, gender, and socioculturally matched peers. A developmental history suggests delayed milestones of development. Parents and teachers may report problems with reasoning, problem-solving, planning, abstract thinking, new learning, and judgment. They may report difficulties in adaptive functioning, which results in failure to meet developmental and sociocultural standards for personal independence and social responsibility. There may be deficits in activities of daily living, communication, social participation, and independent living seen across multiple settings such as home, school, and community.

The diagnosis is based both on clinical assessment and standardized testing of intellectual function. The intelligence quotient (IQ) is less than 70. The deficits can be on a range from borderline and mild problems at one end to severe and profound deficits at the other. The prevalence of intellectual disability is approximately 1% of the general population.

Intellectual disability is a heterogeneous condition with multiple and diverse causes. These may include genetic syndromes and chromosomal abnormalities (e.g. Down syndrome), inborn errors of metabolism, brain malformations, maternal (placental) disease, and environmental influences (e.g. alcohol, drugs, and toxins).

Perinatal causes include a variety of labor and delivery related conditions leading to postnatal encephalopathy. Postnatal causes include hypoxic ischemic injury, traumatic brain injury, infections (e.g. meningitis and encephalitis), demyelinating disorders, seizure disorders, severe and chronic social deprivation, toxic metabolic syndromes, and intoxications (e.g. mercury and lead). The disorder is lifelong and can be influenced by co-occurring conditions such as vision and hearing impairments and epilepsy.

The management of intellectual disability includes detailed clinical assessment, psychometric tests, recognition of underlying causes, exclusion of treatable causes, and symptomatic management. The treatment of comorbidity and the education, training, and support in maximizing the child's potential are crucial. Schooling in regular schools for those with mild disability and special facilities for children with severe disorders is necessary. Parents will also require training and psychosocial support. Rehabilitation programs are mandatory. Such children will benefit from specialist assessment and care.

AUTISM SPECTRUM

The essential features of autism spectrum disorders are persistent impairment in reciprocal social communication and social interaction, restricted and repetitive patterns of behavior, interests, and activities. The inability to hold a normal conversation, initiate social interaction, and failure to respond to social situations is present. Poor eye contact, impaired verbal, and non-verbal communication, deficits in use of gestures, and a lack of facial expression may be present. Difficulties in imaginative play, an absence of interest in friends, and maintaining social relationships is often present.

These abnormalities are also associated with repetitive patterns of behavior, interests, and activities often manifested by stereotyped motor movements and speech, inflexible adherence to routines, ritualized patterns of behavior, and restricted and fixed interests with intense and abnormal focus.

These symptoms start in the early developmental period and cause significant impairment in social, scholastic, and occupational functioning. These are not better explained by intellectual disability.

The prevalence is said to be about 1% of the general population; it is more common in males. The predictive factors of individual outcome are influenced by the presence of intellectual disability, language impairment, and epilepsy.

The management of autism spectrum disorder includes detailed clinical assessment, psychometric tests, and symptomatic management. The treatment of comorbidity and the education, training, and support in maximizing the child's potential are crucial. Schooling in regular schools for those with mild disability and special facilities for children with severe disorders is necessary. Parents will also require training and psychosocial support. Rehabilitation programs are mandatory. These children will benefit from specialist assessment and care.

ATTENTION DEFICIT/HYPERACTIVITY

The essential feature of attention deficit hyperactivity disorder (ADHD) is the persistent pattern of inattention and/or hyperactivity, which interferes within development and functioning. Failure to attend to details, careless mistakes in school work, inability to sustain attention in activities, easy distractibility, difficulty in organizing tasks, reluctance to engage in activities requiring mental effort, and forgetfulness are characteristic of inattention. Hyperactivity is characterized by fidgetiness, inability to sit for still in class, excessive talk, and difficulty waiting for their turn, restlessness, and being always "on the go".

The condition starts before the age of 12 years and is observed across settings such as home, school, and in the community. It clearly interferes with functioning and development. Other mental disorders do not better explain symptoms.

The condition can range from mild to severe. It can be associated with low frustration tolerance, irritability, and lability of mood. About 5% of children are said to have ADHD, and it is more common among boys. The disorder is relatively stable overtime although there can be changes in trajectory.

Children with ADHD may require medication (e.g. methylphenidate and atomoxetine), if the condition is severe. Psychoeducation and support for children and their parents is useful. Behavior and cognitive behavior therapy help many children as do social skills training. Dietary advice and supplements may help. The child will benefit from specialist assessment and care.

STUTTERING

The essential feature of stuttering is a disturbance in the normal fluency and time patterning of speech, which is not appropriate for the child's age. The repetition of sounds and syllables and the prolongation of vowels and consonants, broken words, pauses, and word substitutions may be present. The disturbance causes anxiety about speaking and impairment in effective communication, social participation, and academic difficulties.

The extent of the problems can vary from mild to severe and from situation to situation, often increased in situations of anxiety. The phenomenon may be absent during singing, oral reading, and while talking to pets.

The onset of the problem is in childhood and usually starts by age 6. It may be associated with motor movements (e.g. eye blinks, tics, tremor, and jerking of head).

The majority of children improve with psychoeducation, help, and support. Involvement of families in understanding the nature of the problem is crucial. A reduction of anxiety by reducing demands on the child and slowing down the rate of speech are helpful. An environment free from ridicule is mandatory. Therapy with a speech pathologist is useful. The majority of children seem to recover over time.

Section VI

Basic Issues in Management

23 Basic Psychotropic Medication Management

The commonly employed psychotropic medications, their indications, dose and schedules, route of administration and adverse effects, acute treatment, and prophylaxis are briefly mentioned.

INTRODUCTION

General physicians need to master the basics of employing psychotropic medication in their clinical practice. While there are many different psychotropic drugs available, the repetitive use of a few drugs will allow for increased confidence in their use. Knowing a few drugs, their dosages, schedules, routes of administration, adverse effects, indications, and contraindications will increase confidence and clinical competence. The essential details of antipsychotic and antidepressant medication are given in Tables 23.1 and 23.2, respectively. The principles are briefly highlighted.

CLINICAL EFFICACY

Antipsychotic medication is classified into typical and atypical categories. Despite the reduction and a change in their adverse effects, the efficacy of these drugs is essentially similar. With the exception of clozapine, all antipsychotic medications are equal in their effectiveness in psychosis.

Similarly, antidepressant medication is classified into the traditional tricyclic antidepressants and the newer antidepressants, e.g. selective serotonin reuptake inhibitors (SSRIs). The efficacy of these two classes of medication is equal, with the older drugs having a slight advantage in patients with severe depression.

ADVERSE EFFECT PROFILE

The side-effect profile of the older antipsychotic and antidepressant medication differs markedly from that of the newer drugs. Older medication has more disabling side-effects. Typical antipsychotics cause extra-pyramidal symptoms, sedation, and postural hypotension, while the tricyclic antidepressants cause sedation, postural hypotension and anticholinergic effects.

The newer atypical antipsychotic medications also result in the metabolic syndrome (with an increase in blood sugars and cholesterol). The newer antidepressant, while non-sedating, can cause nausea and gastrointestinal problems.

TABLE 23.1

Antipsychotic Medications, their Adverse Effects, Indications, Dosages, and Duration of Treatment in Primary Care

Medication	Indications	Starting dose/day	Adult dose/day	Common adverse effects	Duration of treatment
Non-sedative oral medication					
Haloperidol	Psychosis without marked agitation	1.5–3 mg	5–10 mg	Tremor, rigidity, bradykinesia, dystonia, akathisia, tardive dyskinesia	At least two years after a first episode of psychosis
Risperidone		1–2 mg	4–6 mg		
Aripiprazole		5 mg	20–30 mg		
Amisulpride		50–100 mg	600–800 mg		Needs to be continued for many years if there is a recurrence or a relapse of symptoms on withdrawal of drug
Ziprasidone		20 mg	100–140 mg		
Sedative oral medication					
Chlorpromazine	Psychosis with marked agitation and sleep disturbance	100–200 mg	600 mg	Tremor, rigidity, bradykinesia, dystonia, akathisia, tardive dyskinesia	
Olanzapine		5 mg	10–15 mg	Sedation, weight gain, elevation of blood sugars and lipids, akathisia	
Intramuscular parenteral medication					
Haloperidol	Psychosis with marked agitation	5 mg	10 mg repeated every hour till patient settles (maximum 30 mg/day)	Sedation, tremor, rigidity, bradykinesia, dystonia, akathisia	
Olanzapine		10 mg	10 mg repeated every hour till patient settles (maximum 20 mg/day)		
Zuclopenthiol		50–150 mg (single dose)	Repeat only after 24 hours; maximum 400 mg over two weeks	Sedation, akathisia	

TABLE 23.1

Antipsychotic Medications, their Adverse Effects, Indications, Dosages, and Duration of Treatment in Primary Care

Medication	Indications	Starting dose/day	Adult dose/day	Common adverse effects	Duration of treatment
Depot intramuscular parenteral medication					
Fluphenazine decanoate	Psychosis with poor medication compliance	25 mg every month	50 mg every month	Tremor, rigidity, bradykinesia, dystonia, akathisia, tardive dyskinesia	
Risperidone microspheres		25 mg every 2 weeks	50 mg every 2 week		
Other medication					
Lorazepam (oral)	Extreme agitation, restlessness	1–2 mg	4–6 mg	Sedation, falls in elderly	Gradually taper within 1–2 weeks
Trihexyphenidyl	Tremor, rigidity, bradykinesia, dystonia, akathisia	2 mg	4–6 mg in divided doses	Dry mouth, constipation, urinary retention	Attempt withdrawal after 3–4 months without symptoms
Promethazine (injection)	For acute dystonia; or along with haloperidol for extreme disturbance	25 mg	25–50 mg	Sedation	Single dose, intramuscular

TABLE 23.2

Antidepressants and Sedative Medications, their Adverse Effects, Indications, Dosages, and Duration of Treatment in Primary Care

Non-sedative antidepressant medication

	Dosage		Adverse effects	Indications	Duration
Fluoxetine	20 mg morning	20 mg for depression and persistent pain; 60 mg for obsessive–compulsive disorder	Nausea, vomiting, diarrhea, restlessness	Unexplained somatic symptoms, depression, panic, phobia, obsessive–compulsive disorder without sleep disturbance	3–6 months followed by a tapering schedule
Sertraline	25 mg morning	50–200 mg per day			
Citalopram	10 mg morning	40 mg per day			
Escitalopram	5 mg morning	20 mg per day			
Paroxetine	10 mg morning	40 mg per day			Can be continued for many years in case of relapse of symptoms on withdrawal

Sedative antidepressant medication

Imipramine, amitriptyline, dothiepin/ dosulepin	25 mg bedtime	50–100 mg	Sedation, dry mouth, constipation, giddiness	Unexplained somatic symptoms, depression, anxiety, panic, phobia associated with disturbed sleep	
Mirtazapine	7.5 mg bedtime	15–30 mg	Sedation, giddiness		

Common sedatives for short-term use

Diazepam	2.5 mg	5–10 mg for sleep; 5–20 mg in divided doses for agitation	Sedation, falls in elderly; potential for addiction	Sleep disturbance, anxiety, agitation	Less than 1 month
Lorazepam	0.5 mg	1–2 mg for sleep: 4–6 mg in divided doses for agitation			

CHOICE OF MEDICATION

As the older and newer classes of antidepressants and antipsychotics are equally efficacious clinically, the choice of medication is often based on matching the symptom profile with the adverse effects of the medication. Patients with insomnia and agitation will benefit from sedative medication, while those without sleep disturbance will prefer non-sedative drugs. Cost is also an issue in resource-poor countries and settings.

COMBATING SIDE-EFFECTS

The older typical antipsychotic medication will require the use of anticholinergic drugs to prevent extra-pyramidal adverse effects (e.g. dystonia, akathisia, and drug-induced parkinsonism). Anticholinergic medication is required as the dose of antipsychotic medication is increased, but may not be necessary for lower doses of the typical drugs and for the newer atypical antipsychotic medication.

DOSE AND SCHEDULES

The principle of starting low and going slow on dose increase is good for practice in primary care. If appropriate, extra medication should be prescribed on an "as needed" or PRN (pro re nata) basis so that the patient and relatives have the option of increasing the dose, if required. Typically, once-a-day schedules are easier to manage, but the dosage can be split into twice a day especially during the initial periods of acute disturbance in psychosis. Antipsychotic medication, and sedative antidepressants, given at bedtime facilitates sleep. The newer antidepressants are taken in the morning as they are non-sedating and may actually cause sleep disturbance, if given at bedtime. Parenteral medication is preferred during acute exacerbations of psychosis and if the patient is violent or if he or she refuses oral medication.

SPECIAL POPULATIONS

Patients with psychiatric presentations secondary to organic and medical conditions, patients with hepatic and renal failure, the elderly, and children will require much smaller doses of medication than healthy adults with similar psychiatric conditions. The policy of starting at a low dose and going up very slowly is necessary in these special populations.

Antipsychotic and antidepressant medication may need to be used in women during pregnancy, but should be employed with caution, and their risks and benefits being discussed in detail with the patient and her family. All drugs may cause problems for the fetus but the experience with the older and typical medications shows that they can be more safely employed in pregnancy. They are to be avoided especially in the first trimester but may be required to prevent disease in those with chronic and recurrent illness. Employing the smallest dose required for prophylaxis is necessary. The use of folic acid to prevent fetal abnormalities should always be considered. Planning for pregnancy in people with chronic and recurrent illness is mandatory. Lithium is best avoided during pregnancy and lactation. The risk of diarrhea with bottle-feeding in low

BOX 23.1 THE POPULARITY OF PILLS

The number of people receiving psychiatric labels and consuming psychotropic medication has increased manifold. This has suggested an increased acceptance of the mental disorder labels and a willingness to consider pills as solutions and wonder drugs. The increasing number of people on medication for mental ill health and claiming disability benefits suggests that an epidemic of mental illness is sweeping the United States of America. Surveys of the general population have suggested that nearly half meet criteria for psychiatric diagnosis.

Many scholars have argued that the "epidemic" is due to expanding diagnostic criteria, which cover every aspect of mental health, distress and illness, medicalizing problems of living rather than an actual increase in mental disease. The nexus between psychiatrists, academia, hospitals, insurance and pharmaceutical industry, which aims to profit and a society looking for quick fixes have been blamed.

and middle-income countries is high, and hence infants can be breastfed even while the mother is on psychotropic medication for most psychotropics (except lithium). The infant should be monitored for excessive sedation and anticholinergic effects such as constipation. Breastfeeding should be timed before the next dose.

MAINTENANCE THERAPY

Antipsychotic medication for acute psychosis should be continued for a period of at least two years to prevent a relapse of the illness. Prophylaxis for much longer periods is required for people with chronic or relapsing disease. The medication should be tapered very gradually as abrupt withdrawal may result in a relapse of the symptoms. The risk of tardive syndromes has to be balanced with the benefits of prophylaxis in the long-term use of antipsychotic medication.

Antidepressant medication should be continued for a year after symptomatic improvement and may be required for a longer term for chronic and relapsing depression. A gradual withdrawal is suggested to assess the need for prophylaxis. Relapses during the gradual withdrawal of medication are often less severe than when medication is abruptly tapered. Such relapses will mandate longer-term prophylaxis.

USE OF BENZODIAZEPINES

While benzodiazepines are powerful medications, their impact on psychosis, depression, and anxiety is limited. They are useful as sedatives and in controlling agitation and violence. However, their potential to lead to dependence and abuse mandates short-term use, and there should be a tapering schedule for their withdrawal. They are best avoided and should be employed with caution. The use of sedative antipsychotics and antidepressant medication in patients with insomnia and agitation will help reduce the need to employ benzodiazepines. Benzodiazepines, when employed, should be tapered and withdrawn within one month.

24 Basic Communication and Counseling Skills

The need for good communication and counseling skills for physicians and health professionals is highlighted. Common errors are mentioned and good techniques described.

INTRODUCTION

A good doctor–patient relationship is the cornerstone of good medical practice. Such relationships, epitomized by physicians with "good bedside manners", contribute to healing. There are many advantages of good communication and counseling skills among physicians and healthcare professionals. Good communication skills contribute to clinical competence, improve diagnostic ability, enhance patient compliance, increase patient satisfaction, and reduce costs.

Nevertheless, many studies suggest that there are serious problems in communication between physicians and their patients in clinical practice. However, training programs rarely address such issues related to communication between physicians and their patients. While the lack of time is often mentioned as a reason for poor communication, it is often due to inadequate training. Poor role models do not help the cause. This chapter briefly discusses the principles of basic communication skills.

WHAT IS THE LACK OF GOOD COMMUNICATION SKILLS ATTRIBUTED TO?

Many reasons, or rather excuses, are often offered for the absence of such skills. The lack of time is a common explanation. The idea that focusing on emotional and psychological issues related to the patient's condition detracts from the task of scientific diagnosis and evidence-based treatments. The fear of causing pain and precipitating emotional reactions in the patient, as breaking bad news causes distress and the possibility that the bearer of bad news is often held responsible for it, also discourages physicians from explaining the issues and helping patients cope with their emotions. Novice physicians are particularly fearful of not knowing all the answers to the patient's questions, of upsetting the medical hierarchy, treading into areas not taught in medical school as well as expressing one's own emotions.

However, while many of these fears are genuine concerns, they can be overcome and the techniques mastered. Investing in communication skills is rewarding both for patients and doctors.

WHAT ARE THE ADVANTAGES OF GOOD COMMUNICATION SKILLS?

Good communication has many advantages and contributes to good doctor–patient relationships. It contributes to the doctor's clinical competence and self-assurance. It increases the efficiency in eliciting relevant information, thereby, improving the doctor's diagnostic ability. Good communication between the physician and the patients improves cooperation during medical and surgical procedures and enhances patient compliance with treatment plans. It reduces patient anxiety and increases patient satisfaction, while reducing cost and improving the utilization of available resources.

Good communication is said to be the cornerstone of good medical practice.

WHAT ARE THE COMMON ERRORS THAT INHIBIT COMMUNICATION?

Doctors with poor communication skills employ "distancing tactics" that inhibit communication (Box 24.1). Such responses often leave the patient stranded and distressed. They take away from the therapeutic relationship. Dismissing the patient's worries or providing immediate and automatic responses to queries rather than exploring the nature and magnitude of the patient's concerns is a common tactic used by doctors with poor communication skills. Such responses are frequently used particularly when the physician is unskilled or does not want to prolong the interaction. Providing false, inappropriate, or premature reassurance without a patient hearing or offering generalizations as soon as the patient mentions his/her fears is also used to not engage with their concerns. "Passing the buck" by asking patients to consult other specialists often leaves the patient stranded. Selectively addressing the patient's physical cues and complaints while neglecting emotional signals and concerns is employed when physicians do not know how to handle emotional issues related to the person's illness. The failure to discuss issues and suggest alternatives disempowers patients and their families.

These responses are usually reflex reactions and inhibit the smooth progression of the interview. A combination of such tactics in a single session can prove disastrous.

WHAT ARE THE BASIC REQUIREMENTS FOR GOOD COMMUNICATION?

The basic requirements, which facilitate good communication, are listed below:

1. *Approach:* The ability to establish a good relationship with patients is important for good doctors. Communication techniques do not work unless the doctor is convinced of their efficacy. Empathy, warmth, respect for, and interest in the patient's welfare are the core of interpersonal skills. Mastering the diverse skills needed to handle different kinds of patients and the variety of situations encountered requires a professional approach.
2. *Environment:* Ensuring privacy encourages disclosure. Using curtains to create an illusion of privacy is useful. Providing comfortable seating, with the patient and the doctor at the same level, aids communication.
3. *Verbal Techniques:* The use of a brief and culturally appropriate greeting at the beginning of the interview is useful (e.g. "Namaste" or "Good morning"). A personal query adds warmth. Asking open-ended questions (e.g. "How are you feeling?")

BOX 24.1 EXAMPLES OF RESPONSES THAT IMPEDE GOOD COMMUNICATION AND THOSE WHICH ENCOURAGE HIGH-QUALITY INTERACTION

1. Dismissing patient's worries –
   Patient: "I am worried that my disease will worsen."
   Doctor (*distancing tactic*): "Don't worry. The medicines will take care of your problem."
   Doctor (*appropriate response*): "Tell me about your worries."
2. Providing false, inappropriate, premature reassurance –
   Patient: "Is there a possibility that some cancer cells may have been left behind after the surgery?"
   Doctor (*distancing tactic*): "The surgery went very well. There is no need to spend time thinking about such things."
   Doctor (*appropriate response*): "While there is a small chance that some cells were left behind, the surgeon felt that he was able to completely remove the tumor as it was small. We plan to give you medication to mop up any remaining malignant cells. We also plan to follow-up regularly to make sure that we pick up the problem early so that we can intervene."
3. Leaving the patient stranded –
   Patient: "My husband does not understand the nature of my disease."
   Doctor (*distancing tactic*): "You will have to explain the details to him."
   Doctor (*appropriate response*): "I am willing to discuss the issues with him. Can you bring him along when you come for your next consultation?"
4. Passing the buck –
   Patient: "I feel tired all the time."
   Doctor (*distancing tactic*): "I think you should talk to your cardiologist about it. He will be able to help."
   Doctor (*appropriate response*): "I will talk to your cardiologist and let you know as to how we can help."
5. Offering generalizations as soon as the patient mentions his/her fears –
   Patient: "I am worried that my condition will not improve."
   Doctor (*distancing tactic*): "Many people have such worries after their first heart attack. These worries will subside."
   Doctor (*appropriate response*): "It is reasonable to have such fears. Tell me more about your concerns and worries."
6. Selective preference for physical cues while neglecting emotional cues –
   Patient: "I am worried about my pain."
   Doctor (*distancing tactic*): "I will prescribe medicine which should relieve the pain."
   Doctor (*appropriate response*): "Tell me about your worry and about your pain."

BOX 24.1   EXAMPLES OF RESPONSES THAT IMPEDE GOOD COMMUNICATION AND THOSE WHICH ENCOURAGE HIGH-QUALITY INTERACTION (*CONTINUED*)

7. Immediate, automatic response without finding out the context, thoughts, feelings, and perceptions –
   Patient: "I have frequent headaches."
   Doctor (*distancing tactic*): "I will prescribe medication for it."
   Doctor (*appropriate response*): "I will discuss the details in a minute, but could you tell me the other problems that you are facing?"

---

allows the patient to present his/her problems and is preferable to closed questions (e.g. "Is the pain better today?"), which tend to bias the reply towards favorable responses.

Allowing the patient time to answer and providing space often helps elicit his/her problems. Picking up verbal cues from the patient and repeating his or her "last three words", or what he/she has just said, will encourage the patient to elaborate his/her thoughts. The use of simple language and avoiding jargon is mandatory. Technical phrases and jargon increase the distance between doctors and their patients, and intimidate, confuse, and reduce the understanding of patients and their relatives about the illness.

4. *Non-verbal Issues:* Leaning forward, maintaining eye contact, nodding appropriately, and listening actively are powerful signals of interest. They are a potent factor in improving the doctor–patient relationship.

WHAT FACTORS ARE ESSENTIAL TO THE SUCCESS OF COUNSELING?

Different schools of psychotherapy argue for and claim superiority of their specific psychotherapeutic techniques. However, there is a growing realization that good psychotherapists and counselors, irrespective of their philosophical approach and psychological orientation, all use certain common techniques that are crucial for psychological improvements in patients. These are listed in Box 24.2.

Factors common to most good counselors include establishing a warm, confiding relationship with the patient. Negative feelings about the patient result in impaired communication. A positive regard for the patient and his/her family is mandatory for psychological intervention and counseling to succeed.

The provision of psychological support to handle the illness and its consequences is necessary. Patients benefit from talking about their problems to their doctors. Allowing time for patients to discuss their concerns is necessary. Exploring emotions is cardinal to success. This allows the physician to gauge the magnitude of the problem, and estimate the gap between the patient's ideas about the illness, its treatment and prognosis, and the actual reality.

Good counselors also need to reorganize the patient's perspectives about his/

BOX 24.2   FACTORS ESSENTIAL FOR THE SUCCESS OF COUNSELING AND PSYCHOLOGICAL INTERVENTION

1. Establish a warm, confiding relationship –
   Example: Show empathy. View the patient's difficulties from the patient's and the family's perspective.
2. Allow time for elaborating issues, raising doubts, expressing feelings –
   Examples: "How are you feeling today?"; "Tell me about your difficulties."; "Do you have any doubts or concerns which you want me to clarify?"
3. Provide psychological support –
   Example: "It must be difficult coping with your symptoms and simultaneously managing your work and home."
4. Reorganize perspectives –
   Examples: "Excessive worry can adversely affect your body and produce distressing symptoms."; "Focusing on the half full glass of water rather than on the fact that it's half empty will reduce distress and improve coping."
5. Arouse hope –
   Example: "I feel that the treatment and your renewed resolve to overcome these difficulties will increase your chances of relief from your symptoms."
6. Transfer responsibility for improvement –
   Example: "While antidepressant medication will help, you will also have to see how you can reduce stress and find new ways to cope with these difficulties. Learning yoga, practicing meditation, and regular physical exercise on a daily basis will help." Prayer and rituals, for those religiously inclined, are also very useful.

---

her illness, providing them with information, clarifying their doubts, and removing misconceptions about their condition. Re-framing and providing an orderly account of the issues is mandatory.

Identifying dysfunctional or harmful patterns of thinking can help patients consider alternative approaches to confronting their problems. Mobilizing disaffection for or creating a sense of dissatisfaction with the patient's present state is necessary for them to be motivated to change their approach. The arousal of hope and the expectation that the distress will reduce, without suggesting unrealistic accounts of the problem, is useful.

Many patients with stress-related problems often shop for miracles from doctors. The responsibility for improvement, when the distress is stress-related, should be gently yet firmly transferred from the doctor to the patient. Patients should be encouraged to use a variety of stress-reduction strategies, including exercise, leisure activities, yoga, meditation, and religion, which should be incorporated into their daily routine.

Patients and relatives should be asked to consider stress in their homes and at work that can contribute to the symptoms and distress. They should be advised to discuss the

BOX 24.3   THE ADVANTAGES OF GOOD COMMUNICATION SKILLS

- Contribute to clinical competence
- Add to physician's self-assurance
- Increase the efficiency in eliciting relevant information
- Improve diagnostic ability
- Improve patient cooperation during medical and surgical procedures
- Enhance patient compliance with treatment plans
- Reduce patient anxiety and increases patient satisfaction
- Reduce costs
- Improve the utilization of available resources

BOX 24.4   THE COMMON MISCONCEPTIONS RELATED TO POOR COMMUNICATION SKILLS AMONG PHYSICIANS

- The lack of time
- The idea that focusing on emotional and psychological issues detracts from the task of diagnosis and treatment
- The fear of causing pain as breaking bad news causes distress
- The fear of being blamed as the bearer of bad news is often held responsible for it
- The fear of precipitating an emotional reaction in the patient
- The fear of not knowing all the answers to the patient's questions
- The fear of upsetting the medical hierarchy
- The fear of treading into areas not taught in medical school
- The fear of expressing one's own emotions

BOX 24.5   THE FALL OF TALKING THERAPIES AND THE RISE OF MIRACLE DRUGS

Despite the fact that talking therapies (e.g. cognitive behavioral therapies, and interpersonal psychotherapy) have been shown to be superior to placebo and equal to medication in many conditions, such as depression and anxiety, the popularity of using psychotropic medications has not diminished. In fact, the ease of use and availability of medication combined with aggressive marketing has resulted in massive profits for pharmaceutical companies. Similarly, despite evidence suggesting that medication effects are overrated for mild to moderate anxiety and depression, and that such conditions benefit from counseling and psychotherapeutic interventions, the popularity of talking therapies have diminished over time.

different solutions possible. Doctors should act only as facilitators and should allow patients to come up with their own solutions for stress.

Attempts to use these techniques when interacting with patients will require a conscious effort at first. However, with practice these techniques will become second nature, and will add to the physician's therapeutic armamentarium.

CONCLUSION

Counseling skills are an essential part of medical practice. These skills can be acquired with practice, and the daily routines of clinicians give ample time for rehearsal. Good communication and counseling skills make a good physician even better.

Physicians should aim to increase their therapeutic armamentarium and their counseling repertoire so that they can manage different kinds of clinical situations, help varied types of people, reduce distinct kinds of distress, and support and improve their coping. Physicians need to not only master the science of disease and cure but also be competent at the art of recognizing distress and providing healing.

25 Problem-solving

Patients who attend primary care with multiple somatic complaints often face stress and problems in their daily life and do not seem to have the ability to resolve conflicts. This chapter briefly explains the problem-solving approach which explores the problem areas, identifies specific problems, considers alternative solutions, and suggests step-wise homework assignments for implementation. It provides ways to monitor progress within the context of a supportive relationship.

INTRODUCTION

Problem-solving is a process that involves identifying the probable causes of a predicament and proposing potential solutions for them. The individual learns skills that he/she can use whenever needed. The patient and doctor together agree on targets and goals, and work towards these in small, specific steps. Such changes in behavior often result in an improvement in the patient's sense of control and well-being. This chapter discusses the steps involved in problem-solving.

EXPLORING STRESS AND COPING

Competent physicians always assess the stress faced by their patients and explore their coping. They are aware of the impact of stress on the etiology of the person's illness, the course and outcome of disease, on treatment compliance, and patient satisfaction. Stress impedes recovery and increases suffering. Patients are often willing to discuss the stress they face with their doctors, provided their physicians show inclination, spend time and are willing to listen to their concerns. Empathy and understanding on part of physicians can result in the early recognition of stressors, the evaluation of the context, and the negotiation of coping strategies, which reduce distress and improve functioning.

EXPLANATION OF THE APPROACH

Discuss the process involved, including the identification of the specific problems that the patient is keen to resolve, searching for specific solutions, and putting these into practice. Introduce the process to the patient with statements such as, "Let us look at ways in which you can handle your stress and deal with your problems."

EXPLORE THE PROBLEM AREAS

Listen carefully to understand the nature of the problems that the patient is experiencing.

Ask questions that encourage him/her to discuss the various difficulties in detail. People facing difficulties often tend to generalize their problems, e.g. a new mother may complain that she is finding motherhood very difficult. Help the patient to break the problem down into specific and workable components, e.g. "After my baby's birth I have no time for my husband or friends. I feel isolated." Ask about specific difficulties in the areas of relationships, employment, finances, housing, legal issues, social isolation, use of alcohol and other drugs, mental health, physical health, sexual adjustment, and bereavement. Summarize the patient's problems as you go along to ensure that you have understood the problem and the patient also feels so.

IDENTIFY A SPECIFIC PROBLEM AND DEFINE GOALS

Start with smaller problems that are most likely to be resolved, such as the issue of social isolation of the new mother, rather than by beginning with discussing more complex issues, such as the patient's relationship with her husband. The goal for this particular problem would be to extend the patient's social network.

EXPLORE ALTERNATIVES AND SOLUTIONS

Consider the steps needed to attain the goal. Put the ball in the patient's court and ask him/her for possible solutions. If the patient finds it difficult to think of possible solutions, encourage him/her to brainstorm and think of any suggestion, no matter how trivial or inappropriate. List out all the solutions and discuss each one's pros and cons. For the new mother with the problem of social isolation, suggestions would include extending her social network and contacting a few friends, her neighbors, or her siblings and parents.

PICK A SOLUTION AND SET THIS AS HOMEWORK

Decide on the solution that fits best. The young mother might choose to phone her old friend as she may feel her brother would be upset on hearing her problems and her neighbors may not be home/have gone away on holiday. Encourage the patient to make specific plans towards the implementation of the goal. The patient in our example was asked when she planned to call her friend, what she would do if the friend was out, etc. Emphasize the need to think and plan ahead and make concrete proposals. Ask the patient what is the worst that could happen with respect to a particular plan. This allows one to get an idea of the sort of fears that the patient may have. It also allows him/her to anticipate a feared situation and plan for all contingencies.

REVIEW PROGRESS DURING SUBSEQUENT SESSIONS

Evaluate how well the patient managed with the planned task. Check the exact details. What did he/she do towards achieving the target? Was it easy or difficult? Do you and the patient agree that the task was done satisfactorily? If the task was done, reinforce the patient and congratulate him/her. The patient can then progress to a new solution towards the same goal or to a solution to a new goal. If the task was partially completed

---

BOX 25.1   STEPS IN PROBLEM-SOLVING

1. Explore context for stress and coping.
2. Listen carefully to understand the nature of the patient's problems.
3. Make a list of problems.
4. Pick out a specific problem worth tackling.
5. Work out goals that the patient would like to set.
6. Consider various solutions and specific steps needed to attain the goal.
7. Review progress; consider other strategies for partially solved issues and choose new goals to be sorted.
8. Consider referral for more complex difficulties.

---

or not attempted, discuss what went wrong and set new goals. Set an alternative, easier task to overcome the problem, and provide encouragement.

CONCLUSION

Problem-solving techniques can often be used to sort out difficulties that people are experiencing. The steps involved include careful listening to understand the nature of the patient's problems, picking out a specific problem worth tackling, working out goals that the patient would like to set, considering various solutions, and practicing the specific steps needed to attain the goal. More complex difficulties and situations may require longer-term therapy or may need to be referred for specialist intervention.

26 Sleep Hygiene

Many patients approach their physician with complaints of poor sleep. A large number of problems related to sleep are consequent to habits that are not compatible with a good night's rest. These require advice regarding alteration in daily patterns and lifestyle that can help to improve sleep. A minority of people have sleep disturbance secondary to its medical or psychiatric causes, which need to be recognized and treated.

INTRODUCTION

Sleep is an important aspect of one's life, which when disturbed can result in significant distress and can alter the ability to function. Many people who present to primary care report problems concerning sleep. This chapter discusses a simple approach to the assessment and management of such patients in primary care and general medical settings.

ASSESSMENT AND MANAGEMENT OF SLEEP DISTURBANCE

Sleep disturbance can be caused by multiple factors, often acting in combination. A systematic and step-wise approach to treating a person with sleep disturbance can help to correctly identify the cause of the problem and to find appropriate solutions.

Medical Causes: Pain, sleep disorders, seizures, and delirium may result in sleep disturbances. These will be evident by taking a careful history and detailed examination. Treatment of the underlying cause will help to improve sleep.

Substance Abuse: Intoxication with substances may result in sleep disturbance. Such patients should be given reassurance and provided safety while waiting for the effects to subside. Withdrawal from substances such as alcohol is associated with significant sleep disturbance. In the immediate withdrawal period, benzodiazepines may be prescribed in a tapering schedule. If sleep disturbance persists after the benzodiazepines are tapered and stopped, a low-dose antidepressant may be used. If the withdrawal is associated with psychosis, low-dose antipsychotic medication is necessary.

Medication Adverse Effects: Prescribed medication may have side-effects that interfere with sleep. For example, antipsychotic medication can result in akathisia or a sense of restlessness and an inability to remain still. Such adverse effects will require a reduction in the dose of the offending agent, if possible, along with symptomatic management. The addition of low dose of benzodiazepines, such as lorazepam, will reduce the akithisia and improve sleep.

Psychiatric Disorders: Depression, anxiety, and psychosis interfere with sleep. Management with sedative antidepressants, anxiolytics, or antipsychotic agents may be required. However, long-term use of benzodiazepines should be avoided as they can lead to dependence.

Psychosocial Stress: Events in the environment and anxiety related to daily stress can result in anxiety and disturbed sleep. Problem-solving techniques need to be employed to deal with the problem. In addition, learning relaxation strategies and practicing deep breathing exercises can help to reduce anxiety.

Environmental Factors: Attempting to sleep in an area that is noisy or trying to sleep on uncomfortable bedding can interfere with sleep. Individual aspects of the environment need to be rectified.

Poor Sleep Hygiene: Certain patterns or habits can prevent an individual from having a refreshing sleep. Sleep hygiene is a variety of different practices that are necessary to have normal, quality nighttime sleep and full daytime alertness:

- Ensure that the bedroom environment is conducive to sleep. It should be quiet, comfortable, and free from light. It should not be used for activities other than sleep (and sex, if applicable).
- Do not watch television or read while lying in bed. This helps to associate your bed with sleep.
- Maintain a comfortable temperature in the bedroom so that you are not required to awaken at night to open or to close windows, turn on fans, etc.
- If you are in bed but cannot get to sleep, turn on the light, leave the bed and do

---

BOX 26.1   SLEEP HYGIENE

The first intervention for sleep problems should include sleep hygiene techniques:
- Bedroom environment is quiet, comfortable, free from light and conducive to sleep.
- The bed should not be used for activities other than sleep (e.g. watching television or reading while lying in bed).
- Maintain a comfortable temperature in the bedroom.
- If you are in bed but cannot get to sleep, leave the bed and do something different until you feel sleepy.
- Avoid caffeine, alcohol, and tobacco in the evenings and night.
- Avoid large and spicy meals just before going to bed; also do not go to bed hungry.
- Avoid excessive liquids in the evening to will minimize the need for nighttime trips to the bathroom.
- Wake up at the same time every day.
- Do not take naps during the day.
- A regular exercise program in the morning or afternoon can help to promote sleep. Avoid vigorous exercise at least 3 hours of bedtime.

something different like reading a book. Do not engage in stimulating activity. Return to bed only when you feel sleepy.
- Avoid caffeine, alcohol, and tobacco in the evenings and night.
- Avoid large and spicy meals just before going to bed. On the other hand, do not go to bed hungry.
- Avoid excessive liquids in the evening. Reducing liquid intake will minimize the need for nighttime trips to the bathroom.
- Wake up at the same time every day, even on weekends, no matter how little you slept. A regular wake time in the morning leads to regular times of sleep onset, and helps to set your biological clock.
- Do not take naps during the day. This can disturb the normal pattern of sleep and wakefulness.
- A regular exercise program in the morning or afternoon can help to promote sleep. Vigorous exercise should not occur within 3 hours of when you intend to go to bed.

Sleep disturbances and daytime sleepiness are the most telling signs of poor sleep hygiene. If a patient describes a sleep problem, his or her sleep routine needs to be evaluated and the necessary alterations need to be made to ensure adequate sleep.

Section VII

Appendix:
Information Leaflets

a. Dementia

b. Alcohol Dependence

c. Acute Psychosis

d. Chronic Psychosis and Schizophrenia

e. Bipolar Disorder

f. Depression and Anxiety

g. Persistent Physical Symptoms and Anxiety about Health

h. Marriage and the Law

i. Making a WILL

a. Information leaflet on dementia for patients and their families

WHAT IS DEMENTIA?

Dementia is a general progressive deterioration in memory and thinking, caused by several different types of brain disease. It affects mainly older people, usually aged over 65 years. As the brain is important for everything that we do (remembering, talking, working things out, planning, and making choices), older people with dementia become more and more disabled, and need more and more help and support, even with simple tasks.

WHAT ARE THE SYMPTOMS OF DEMENTIA?

Dementia results in impairment of multiple domains of brain function.
- The central feature is problems with memory. There is an inability to learn new information and a tendency to forget previously learned information. While occasional memory failings are normal, memory problems are likely to be significant if they happen regularly, and if the problems seem to be getting worse. Memory problems include:
- Forgetting
  - Recent events (e.g. cannot remember what they were told yesterday, recent visits by relatives, and festivals)
  - Daily activities (e.g. cannot remember where they kept the keys, and money)
  - Cooking (e.g. often forget to add salt or some other commonly used ingredient to the food)
  - Shopping (e.g. frequently forget to bring back the required items, and are not able to get back the correct change)
  - Going out of the house (e.g. getting lost when out of the house)
  - Paying bills (e.g. cannot remember if they have paid bills)
- Worsening of speech and use of language over time – for example, forgetting the names of close friends and relatives, forgetting the names of familiar objects (e.g. watch, pen, and spoon), difficulty in understanding simple instructions, difficulty in holding a conversation, or decline in the amount or quality of conversation. Later they may find it difficult to communicate their desires and needs.
- Inability to carry out simple actions despite normal movement of limbs – for example, difficulty in dressing, difficulty in combing hair, or difficulty in brushing teeth.

217

- Difficulty in recognizing familiar objects or people despite normal eyesight – for example, problems in recognizing chair, watch, pen, spoon; and problems in recognizing family members.
- Difficulty in planning and carrying out a complex activity – for example, difficulty in shopping, going to the post office, or going to a town nearby.

The impairment occurs in multiple areas, and causes a significant decline in functioning compared to past performance, including significant impediment in social and occupational functioning.

The following behavioral and psychological symptoms may occur in more advanced dementia:

- Feeling that people are stealing their belongings and will harm them
- Hallucinations (hearing voices of strange people)
- Getting very angry and violent without provocation
- Feeling very sad, depressed, and crying without reason
- Anxiety, repeated questioning
- Incontinence (of bladder and/or bowel)
- Apathy and loss of interest in surroundings
- Dis-inhibited and inappropriate behavior
- Disturbed sleep at night
- Wandering and getting lost
- Being confined to the bed

Dementia should be differentiated from other conditions

Dementia differs from age-related cognitive decline and a condition called mild cognitive impairment (MCI), in which there is significant memory impairment in the absence of other cognitive deficits, but which results in social or occupational dysfunction.

WHAT ARE THE CAUSES OF DEMENTIA?

There are many causes of dementia. All of them are due to diseases of the brain. Dementia can also run in families. There are also reversible causes of dementia that your doctor will attempt to exclude through blood tests and brain scans. Medical conditions such as high blood pressure, uncontrolled diabetes, high cholesterol, smoking, drinking, and being overweight can increase the risk of dementia, and need to be controlled.

WHAT ARE THE COMMON LOCAL BELIEFS ABOUT CAUSATION?

Many people believe that dementia is a part of normal aging, which needs to be accepted. Supernatural causes such as karma, black magic, evil spirits, sin, and punishment by God are also suggested as causal. It is not the aim of this leaflet to dismiss such beliefs about causation. This leaflet aims to present a medical view of the condition. People seem to hold more than one belief about the cause. While we do not ask you to abandon your cultural beliefs, we would suggest that you also consider a medical model for dementia. Other treatments from traditional and faith healers and shamans can be employed in combination with medical and psychosocial treatment.

WHAT IS THE TREATMENT FOR DEMENTIA?

The main treatment for delaying the progress of the disease comprises drugs that inhibit the enzyme acetylcholine esterase. Newer drugs that act on other receptors are also available. However, all these medications cannot reverse the process and have to be taken for a long time.

Specific drugs (e.g. antipsychotics and antidepressants) can help manage the symptoms of sleep disturbance, depression, restlessness, psychosis, and other behavioral and psychological symptoms of dementia.

Many of the risk factors (diabetes, hypertension, increased cholesterol, etc.) will need to be controlled. You should ask your doctor about these.

WHAT CAN THE PATIENT AND RELATIVES DO TO DELAY THE PROCESS AND IMPROVE COPING?

The following simple measures can help in coping with dementia and prevent/delay the onset of dementia in the elderly:

- *Taking notes:* Taking notes and writing down messages are of help.
- *Being organized:* Being tidy and organized will allow you to remember where you have put things. A regular routine will help you remember what you are supposed to be doing.
- *Using a diary:* Keeping a diary of activities will help in recall. Similarly, keeping a diary for appointments will help keep up with daily tasks.
- *Keeping fit:* Getting regular exercise, eating and drinking moderately, and not smoking will keep you healthy. The use of proper spectacles and hearing aids will improve vision and hearing, and help with remembering.
- *Regular health checks:* Early detection and treatment of diseases will help prevent worsening of dementia.
- *Use your mind:* Hobbies such as doing quizzes, crosswords, reading, learning passages or poems, and card games, may help to offset the effects of aging.
- *Reality orientation* is a means of helping people with dementia remember where they are, the day, date and time, and what is happening. This is done by constantly telling them these things and getting them to repeat what they have been told.
- *Mnemonics* are tricks to help us memorize particular things. For example, the rhyme "30 days hath September" – for remembering the lengths of the months.
- *External aids:* Calendars, clocks, lists and diaries are of help.

The following strategies will help people with dementia:

- *A regular and structured routine:* Following a simple yet regular daily and weekly routine helps maintain orientation.
- *Labeling or color coding:* This is useful in the case of objects such as switches, files, books, shelves, and containers.
- *Avoiding unfamiliar activities or new situations:* This prevents confusion and disorientation.

- *Helpful tips:* Many specific tips to manage issues related to people with dementia can be found on the net. For example, Alzheimer Disease International has a very helpful website for caregivers. (http://www.alz.co.uk/carers/).

WHAT IS THE CLINICAL OUTCOME FOR PEOPLE WITH DEMENTIA?

Most dementias result in a progression of the disease. The medication and psychosocial treatment strategies currently available delay the progression of the disease but cannot prevent the slow decline in functioning.

You can discuss these and other issues with your doctor, nurse, or occupational therapist. You should feel free to clarify any doubts you have about dementia and its treatment.

b. Information leaflet for patients with alcohol problems and for their families

WHEN DOES ALCOHOL USE BECOME A PROBLEM?

Alcohol use becomes a problem when it harms the person's health or interferes with his work and family life. Persistence of problem drinking usually leads to a dependence pattern.

WHAT ARE THE SYMPTOMS OF ALCOHOL DEPENDENCE?

The symptoms of dependence on alcohol include many of the following: (i) withdrawal symptoms (difficulty with sleep, tremors, irritability, restlessness, etc.) upon not taking alcohol; (ii) increased tolerance (increased consumption of alcohol to get the same effect); (iii) greater concern with obtaining alcohol than with daily chores; (iv) strong desire to use alcohol nearly every day; (v) unable to cut down the amount of alcohol consumed; (vi) problems at work (e.g. frequent absenteeism); (vii) impairment in family and social roles.

WHAT ARE THE COMMON MEDICAL PROBLEMS DUE TO EXCESSIVE CONSUMPTION OF ALCOHOL?

Excessive use of alcohol can result in impairment of and damage to many systems of the body. Impairment of liver functions occurs with excessive and regular use of alcohol. Increased liver enzymes, jaundice, liver enlargement, and finally shrinkage (cirrhosis) of the liver, and coma occur with persistent excessive use. Vomiting blood or passing blood in stool are signs of damage to the stomach and intestines. Severe abdominal pain usually results from damage to the pancreas. Damage to the brain usually results in episodes of confusion, seizures, memory impairment, difficulty in walking, and dementia. The persistent use of alcohol also results in psychiatric problems such as fear, disorientation, feeling that other people will harm/kill the person, "hearing voices", depression, and anxiety. Sexual dysfunction is also common with prolonged use of alcohol.

WHAT ARE THE EFFECTS OF ALCOHOL PROBLEMS ON THE FAMILY?

Family members of people with alcohol problems can feel frustrated, hurt, and angry if their advice is not accepted. They can be concerned about the person's safety and well-being, and worried about the future, but may be unsure about how to help. They may be concerned about the effects on the rest of the family and worried about the financial consequences. Alcohol problems often result in breakdown in family communication and put family members under severe stress. It is often useful to talk about these issues with family and friends who will be understanding and supportive. Involving the elders in the family may be an option for some. Reporting to the local panchayat or the women's police station in extreme situations in which physical abuse is present may also be helpful. You should feel free to discuss these and other issues with your doctor or the doctor who is treating your family member for alcohol problems.

WHAT ARE THE TREATMENTS FOR ALCOHOL PROBLEMS?

The goal of treatment ranges from getting the patient to control consumption to helping him give up drinking alcohol completely. While abstinence is the preferred goal, a marked reduction in intake is preferable to continued intake of alcohol at the present level that is causing problems. The treatment can be divided into two phases: (i) detoxification and (ii) de-addiction.

Detoxification: The detoxification phase of treatment involves the following: (i) assessment of the problem drinking; (ii) diagnosis and management of nutritional deficiencies; (iii) diagnosis and management of the physical and psychiatric complications of alcohol; (iv) stopping alcohol intake completely and substituting it with medication (e.g. diazepam and chlordiazepoxide); and (v) assessing and improving motivation to stop alcohol use.

Detoxification can be either home-based or part of a hospital program. A hospital-based program is preferable when the addiction is severe, the person has physical and psychiatric complications due to prolonged use of alcohol, or if the home-based approach has failed. This phase of treatment usually takes 7–10 days.

De-addiction program: Psychological treatments are important to prevent the relapse of alcohol use after detoxification. These include an analysis of behavior, the identification of cues which result in alcohol use, and their substitution with healthy behaviors. De-addiction programs also include training of people with poor social skills and the lack of assertiveness. These therapies manage issues related to interpersonal, marital, and family conflicts as well. Problems at work and finding solutions to them also figure in the therapy. People are helped with their stress and adjustment difficulties. Sexual dysfunction secondary to alcohol use is also treated.

The de-addiction package also includes medication that reduces craving (e.g. acamprosate) or limits the effects of alcohol (e.g. naltrexone). Medication that produces serious adverse reactions (e.g. disulfiram) is also employed in treatment and the fear of the serious consequences keeps many people away from drinking alcohol.

HOW EFFECTIVE IS THE THERAPY?

Excessive consumption of alcohol is a habit that needs to be broken. The person's motivation and resolve to stop drinking alcohol is the most important predictor of abstinence. The therapy will help people who want to give up the habit. While many people are able to abstain from alcohol for significant periods of time after the detoxification and de-addiction program, others are able to reduce the amount consumed. Some continue to use alcohol without any reduction. A relapse of drinking after a period of abstinence can also occur. People with alcohol problems are encouraged to come back for treatment if they resume drinking or if they are unable to stop or change their habit. The doctors, nurses, and therapists will again try and help them overcome their habit. Repeated detoxification and repeated de-addiction treatments may be necessary for some people before they are able to give up the habit. Re-admission for detoxification and de-addiction may also be useful when frequent or prolonged relapses occur.

As with all habits, giving up the habit of drinking is not an easy task. Giving up alcohol for a certain length of time, especially after medical detoxification, is easy. However, abstaining from alcohol is the main challenge. The main ingredients for success are a change in the person's attitude, philosophy, and lifestyle. Such a change will allow the person to cope with the day-to-day stress, frustrations, and problems in life without resorting to the use of alcohol.

FOLLOW-UP AND BOOSTER SESSION

Follow-up and booster sessions with the doctor or therapist after discharge from hospital and at regular intervals may increase the person's resolve and resources to remain abstinent for long periods of time.

You can discuss these and other issues with your doctor, nurse, or occupational therapist. You should feel free to clarify any doubts you have about the alcohol problem and its treatment.

C. Information leaflet on acute psychosis for patients and their families

WHAT IS ACUTE PSYCHOSIS?

Acute psychosis is a mental illness due to disease of the brain. It is sudden in onset and typically of short duration, about one month. It can occur in any age group, but is often seen between the ages 15 and 40 years.

WHAT ARE THE SYMPTOMS OF ACUTE PSYCHOSIS?

The symptoms of acute psychosis include abnormal beliefs (delusions) and hearing voices or seeing visions (hallucinations), and may involve abnormal behavior.

A delusion is a belief that is held with complete conviction. However, it is based on a misinterpretation or misunderstanding of situations or events. Other people usually see such beliefs as mistaken, strange, or unrealistic. The person may believe that he/she is being persecuted, that he/she has special powers, that his/her spouse is unfaithful, or that he/she is being controlled or being talked about by strangers. The person may or may not act on such beliefs.

A hallucination occurs when you hear, smell, feel or see something that is not actually there. "Hearing voices" and "seeing visions" of people who are not there is common. The voices and visions appear to be coming from outside, are clear, and appear very real. The voices can be pleasant, but are often rude or abusive. Occasionally, the voices command the person to do things or perform actions. However, they can often be ignored. Other positive symptoms include muddled thinking, sleep disturbance, and restlessness.

Abnormal behavior may involve severe agitation, restlessness, wandering, preoccupation, social isolation, and withdrawal. Sleep disturbance and fear are also common. The person may also report loss of appetite, the lack of motivation to work, and difficulty in concentrating on daily chores.

People with the disorder may not acknowledge the presence of a mental illness and may refuse treatment.

WHAT CAUSES ACUTE PSYCHOSIS?

The causes of the disease are not very clear. It is likely to be a combination of several different factors, which will be different for different people. The disease can run in families and may be transmitted through genes. Brain damage during birth or viral infections during pregnancy can also contribute. Cannabis (*ganja*) and alcohol can precipitate or worsen the disease. Psychological stress at work and in the family can increase the risk of developing the disease.

WHAT ARE THE COMMON LOCAL BELIEFS ABOUT CAUSATION?

Many people in India believe that mental illness is caused by supernatural forces. Karma, black magic, evil spirits, sin, and punishment by God, among other things, have been suggested as causes for the illness. Such explanations are also accepted by many religions and cultures. Many people seem to simultaneously hold more than one belief about the nature and cause of mental illness. The belief that it arises from a disease seems to be held with equal conviction as are beliefs about its being a supernatural phenomenon.

It is not the aim of this leaflet to dismiss such beliefs about causation. This leaflet aims to present a medical view of the condition. People are free to hold more than one belief about the cause. While we do not ask you to abandon your cultural beliefs about the illness, we would suggest that you also consider the disease model for the illness. The medications used in the treatment of the condition seem to have a powerful impact on the outcome of the illness and can be combined with other views on causation. Other treatments from traditional and faith healers and *shamans* can be employed in combination for the relief of suffering.

WHAT IS THE CLINICAL OUTCOME FOR PEOPLE WITH ACUTE PSYCHOSIS?

Many people with this condition do well with medication and treatment. Many do not have to get admitted to the hospital, and two out of three people are able to settle down, work, get married, and lead a normal life.

WHAT WILL HAPPEN WITHOUT TREATMENT?

Many symptoms, such as hearing voices and holding strange beliefs, can be distressing for the person and the family. Depression and suicide are more common in people with acute psychosis. Research suggests that the longer the condition is left untreated, the greater is its impact on the person's life. The sooner it is identified and treated, the better the outlook. While some people may recover from the illness, others may have a more chronic course.

WHAT IS THE TREATMENT FOR THE DISEASE?

Medication should be started as soon as possible and will reduce the most disturbing symptoms of the illness. However, it does not provide a complete answer. Support from the family and friends, psychological treatment, and employment are also equally important. The majority of people with the disease can receive treatment while living at home, although a small proportion may have to be admitted to hospital for a few weeks to initiate treatment.

Medication for acute psychosis, called antipsychotics, comes in the form of tablets, capsules or syrup. These include "first-generation" (also called typical) drugs, such as chlorpromazine and haloperidol. These drugs act on a chemical messenger in the brain called dopamine. The side-effects of these drugs include tremors of the hands, stiffness of the limbs, restlessness, and sexual dysfunction. Some of these side-effects can be prevented by taking anticholinergic medication (e.g. trihexyphenidyl). About 1 in 20 people who take this medicine for long periods may develop a long-term side-effect called tardive dyskinesia. It includes persistent movements, usually of the mouth and tongue.

Several newer medications have been available over the past 10 years. They work on a different range of chemical messengers in the brain (e.g. serotonin) and are called "atypical" or "second-generation" antipsychotics (e.g. risperidone, olanzapine, and quetiapine). Although they are less likely to cause tremors, stiffness, and restlessness, they may cause weight gain and problems with sexual function. They also seem much less likely to produce tardive dyskinesia. Many people who use these newer medications have found the side-effects less troublesome than those of the older medications.

Antipsychotic medications work well for many people – about 4 in 5 people are helped with them. The medications will have to be taken for 1–2 years after an episode of acute psychosis. A relapse of symptoms is much less likely to occur during this period if the medication is continued, even when the patient feels well.

Electroconvulsive therapy can also be employed for a severe episode of acute psychosis, especially when the person risks harming himself or others.

Psychological treatments include education about the illness and its treatment, counseling, supportive psychotherapy, cognitive behavioral therapy, and family therapy. It is important that the patient be supervised. It is often not useful to argue with the patient's beliefs, though they may be wrong. Confrontation should be avoided unless it is necessary to prevent harmful or disruptive behavior. The patient should be encouraged to maintain his or her daily routine of activities. Chores should be broken into smaller steps. Offering rewards and praise, even if tasks are not perfectly done, will help. Encouraging re-entry into work when possible is advisable. It is also important to ensure that excessive demands are not made of the patient, as this could be detrimental to the progress and may precipitate a relapse. Recovery often takes place in small steps. Your doctor, psychiatrist, clinical psychologist, social worker, psychiatric nurse, or occupational therapist will discuss the issues with you.

How long will I have to take medication?

Most psychiatrists will suggest that you take medication for many months. For example, if you have been suffering from the disease for one month, you will have to take medication for about two years. If you want to reduce or stop the medication, it should be discussed with your doctor. The medication should be reduced gradually so that it can be increased if any symptoms return and you become unwell again. In case there is a relapse of the disease on reducing medicines, the medication must be continued for a longer period.

Getting back to normal

Acute psychosis generally has a good outcome, with many people returning to normal lives without any relapse of the illness. However, in a minority of people, the illness can recur or can become chronic. Relapse of the illness can be managed with medication and with psychological treatments and rehabilitation.

You can discuss these and other issues with your doctor, nurse, or occupational therapist. You should feel free to clarify any doubts you have about the illness and its treatment.

d. Information leaflet on chronic psychosis and schizophrenia for patients and their families

WHAT IS SCHIZOPHRENIA?

Schizophrenia is a mental illness due to disease of the brain. It affects around 1 in every 100 people and affects men and women equally. It usually occurs between the ages 15 and 40 years.

WHAT ARE THE SYMPTOMS OF SCHIZOPHRENIA?

The symptoms of schizophrenia can be grouped as positive and negative. The "positive symptoms" include abnormal beliefs (delusions) and "hearing voices" or "seeing visions" (hallucinations), and may involve abnormal behavior.

A delusion is a belief that is held with complete conviction. However, it is based on a misinterpretation or misunderstanding of situations or events. Other people usually see such beliefs as mistaken, strange, or unrealistic. Such beliefs may involve feelings of being persecuted, of having special powers, of infidelity on the part of one's spouse, of being controlled, or of being talked about by strangers. The person may or may not act on such beliefs.

A hallucination occurs when you hear, smell, feel, or see something that is not actually there. "Hearing voices" and "seeing visions" of people who are not there is common. The voices and visions appear to be coming from outside, are clear, and appear very real. The voices can be pleasant, but are often rude or abusive. Occasionally, the voices command the person to do things or perform actions. However, they can often be ignored. Other positive symptoms include muddled thinking, sleep disturbance, and restlessness.

The "negative symptoms" include lack of energy to perform daily chores, the lack of motivation to work, and difficulty with concentration. While these symptoms may not be prominent, they are equally disabling.

People with the disorder may not acknowledge the presence of a mental illness and may refuse treatment.

WHAT CAUSES SCHIZOPHRENIA?

The causes of the disease are not very clear. It is likely to be a combination of several different factors that will be different for different people. The disease can run in families and may be transmitted through genes. Brain damage during birth or viral

228

infections during pregnancy can also contribute. Cannabis (*ganja*) and alcohol can precipitate or worsen the disease. Psychological stress at work and in the family can increase the risk of developing the disease.

WHAT ARE THE COMMON LOCAL BELIEFS ABOUT CAUSATION?

Many people in India believe that mental illness, including schizophrenia, is caused by supernatural forces. Karma, black magic, evil spirits, sin, and punishment by God, among other things, have been suggested as the cause for the illness. Such explanations are also accepted by many religions and cultures. Many people seem to simultaneously hold more than one belief about the nature and cause of mental illness. The belief that the illness arises from a disease seems to be held with equal conviction as beliefs of supernatural causation.

It is not the aim of this leaflet to dismiss such beliefs about causation. This leaflet aims to present a medical view of the condition. People are free to hold more than one belief about the cause. While we do not ask you to abandon your cultural belief about the illness, we would suggest that you also consider the disease model for the illness. The medications used in the treatment of the condition seem to have a powerful impact on the outcome of the illness and can be combined with other views on causation. Other treatments from traditional and faith healers and shamans can be employed in combination for the relief of suffering.

WHAT IS THE CLINICAL OUTCOME FOR PEOPLE WITH SCHIZOPHRENIA?

Many people with the condition do well with medication and treatment. Many do not have to get admitted to hospital, and two out of every three people are able to settle down, work, get married, and lead a normal life.

WHAT WILL HAPPEN WITHOUT TREATMENT?

Many symptoms, such as hearing voices and holding strange beliefs, can be distressing for the person and the family. Depression and suicide are more common in people with schizophrenia. Research suggests that the longer schizophrenia is left untreated, the greater is its impact on the person's life. The sooner it is identified and treated, the better the outlook.

WHAT IS THE TREATMENT FOR THE DISEASE?

Medication should be started as soon as possible and will reduce the most disturbing symptoms of the illness. However, it does not provide a complete answer. Support from family and friends, psychological treatment, and employment are also equally important. The majority of people with the disease can receive treatment while living at home, although a small proportion may have to be admitted to the hospital for a few weeks to initiate treatment.

Medication for schizophrenia, called antipsychotics, come in the form of tablets, capsules, or syrup. These include "first-generation" (also called typical) drugs, such as chlorpromazine and haloperidol. These medications can also be given as a weekly or monthly injection. These drugs act on a chemical messenger in the brain called dopamine. The side-effects of these drugs include tremors of the hands, stiffness of the limbs, restlessness, and sexual dysfunction. Some of these side-effects can be prevented by taking anticholinergic medication (e.g. trihexyphenidyl). About 1 in 20 people who take this medicine for long periods may develop a long-term side-effect called tardive dyskinesia. This includes persistent movements, usually of the mouth and tongue.

Several newer medications have been available over the past 10 years. They work on a different range of chemical messengers in the brain (e.g. serotonin) and are called "atypical" or "second-generation" antipsychotics (e.g. risperidone, olanzapine, quetiapine, and clozapine). They may also help the negative symptoms, on which the older drugs have very little effect. Although they are less likely to cause tremors, stiffness, and restlessness, they may cause weight gain and problems with sexual function. They also seem much less likely to produce tardive dyskinesia. Many people who use these newer medications have found the side-effects less troublesome than those of the older medications.

Antipsychotic medications work well for many people – about four in five people get help from them. They control the disorder, but do not cure it. The medications will have to be taken for long periods in order to prevent the symptoms from returning. This is much less likely to happen if the medication is continued even when the patient feels well.

Electroconvulsive therapy can also be employed for severe episodes of the disorder especially when the person risks harming himself or others.

Psychological treatments include education about the illness and its treatment, counseling and supportive psychotherapy, cognitive behavioral therapy, and family therapy. It is important that the patient be supervised. It is often not useful to argue with the patient's beliefs, though they may be wrong. Confrontation should be avoided unless it is necessary to prevent harmful or disruptive behavior. The patient should be encouraged to maintain his or her daily routine of activities. Chores should be broken into smaller steps. Offering rewards and praise, even if tasks are not perfectly done, will help. Re-entry into work, when possible, should be encouraged. It is also important to ensure that excessive demands are not made of the patient, as this could be detrimental to progress and may precipitate a relapse. Recovery often takes place in small steps. Your psychiatrist, clinical psychologist, social worker, psychiatric nurse, or occupational therapist will discuss the issues with you.

How long will I have to take medication?

Most psychiatrists will suggest that you take medication for many months. For example, if you have been suffering from the disease for two months you will have to take medication for about two years. If you want to reduce or stop the medication, it should be discussed with your doctor. The medication should be reduced gradually so that it can be increased if any symptoms return and you become unwell again. In case there is a relapse of the disease on reducing medicines, the medication must be continued for a longer period.

GETTING BACK TO NORMAL

Schizophrenia can make it difficult to deal with the demands of everyday life even after the symptoms are controlled. Sometimes, this is because of the symptoms. Sometimes, the illness may have gone on for so long that the person may have got out of the habit of doing things for him/herself. It can be difficult to get back to doing ordinary things, such as washing, shopping, making a phone call, or chatting with a friend. These problems can be managed with psychological treatments and rehabilitation.

You can discuss these and other issues with your doctor, nurse, or occupational therapist. You should feel free to clarify any doubts you have about the illness and its treatment.

e. Information leaflet on bipolar disorder for patients and their families

WHAT IS BIPOLAR DISORDER?

Bipolar disorder is characterized by mood swings, or episodes that are far beyond what most people experience in their lives. These episodes consist of (i) low mood, i.e. feelings of intense depression and despair, called "depression" and (ii) high mood, i.e. feelings of elation and restlessness, called "mania". The condition used to be called "manic depression". Most people usually experience both depressive and manic episodes.

WHAT ARE THE SYMPTOMS OF BIPOLAR DISORDER?

The disorder usually starts in the late teens or early twenties. It affects both men and women equally. The depressive episodes are characterized by sadness, low mood, crying spells, preoccupation, social withdrawal, lack of confidence, restlessness, sleep disturbance, loss of appetite, difficulty in concentration, poor work performance, and suicidal ideation. The symptoms of the manic episodes include elation, excessive happiness, making unrealistic plans, feeling of increased energy, spending a lot of money, difficulty with concentration, poor work performance, irritability, anger, sleep disturbance, and decreased appetite. Occasionally, people with the disorder can hear "voices" during episodes of depression or mania.

These episodes usually last a few weeks to a few months and can be very disruptive. They can subside spontaneously but have a propensity to recur. While many people with the disorder may return to normal levels of function, some can have persistent depression or difficulty at home or with work.

WHAT ARE THE CAUSES OF BIPOLAR DISORDER?

The disorder is a disease of the brain. While the episodes can be precipitated by stressful life experiences, they often have a genetic basis and can run in families.

WHAT IS THE TREATMENT FOR THE DISORDER?

The treatment includes (i) treatment of the manic or depressive episodes and (ii) the prevention of future episodes (prophylaxis). Medication and psychological therapies are useful and are briefly mentioned.

Medication: Medication is useful in preventing future episodes of illness and in hastening recovery from episodes of mania and depression. Lithium, carbamazepine, and sodium valproate are mood stabilizers and are used to prevent the recurrence of illness. They are also useful in hastening recovery from episodes of mania and depression. These drugs will have to be taken for a long time when employed for prevention of the disease. The common adverse effects of lithium are increased thirst, weight gain, and a tendency to pass more urine than usual. The common adverse effects of carbamazepine and valproate include sedation, nausea, and weight gain. The dosage of these medications is adjusted on the basis of clinical response and on blood levels. Yearly blood tests to check for renal, thyroid, and liver functions are required for those taking these medications for long-term prophylaxis. The blood levels have to be monitored regularly as patients can develop severe symptoms if the levels are above the recommended range (e.g. vomiting, diarrhea, blurred vision, confusion, and difficulty in walking). The dosage will need to be reduced or the tablets temporarily stopped if such symptoms develop.

Mood stabilizers can be started if the episode of depression or mania is severe and disruptive. They need to be prescribed if the patient has suffered from many episodes of illness. They should be continued for two years if started after the first episode of illness and much longer if prescribed for prophylaxis.

Antidepressant medications can be used if the depressive episodes are severe and are usually given under the cover of a mood stabilizer. The newer antidepressants (SSRIs) are preferred to the older tricyclic antidepressants. Antidepressants need to be continued for at least eight weeks after recovery from the depressive episode. They need to be tapered and withdrawn slowly. The common adverse effects of SSRIs include nausea and restlessness. Antidepressants should be discontinued if the person switches/has switched to mania while on such treatment.

Antipsychotic medication is employed for mania. The newer antipsychotic drugs (e.g. risperidone and olanzapine) are preferred to the older drugs, which have disabling adverse effects (stiffness, tremor, slowness of movements, etc.). These need to be withdrawn gradually after the manic symptoms have remitted.

In case women on these medications are planning to get pregnant, they should discuss the issues with their doctor and weigh the risk of relapse against the risk of problems for the fetus. Older or typical antipsychotic medication and carbamazepine are the preferred drugs during pregnancy. The cost in terms of risk to the fetus should be balanced against the benefits of prophylaxis.

Electroconvulsive therapy can also be employed for severe episodes of the disorder, especially when the person risks harming himself or others.

Psychological treatments: Psychological treatment includes psychoeducation about the illness and its treatment, monitoring of mood, discussion of general coping strategies, and cognitive behavior therapy for depression. Stress related to home, relationships, and work also needs to be discussed.

ADVICE FOR FAMILY AND FRIENDS

Episodes of mania or depression can be very distressing for family and friends. Depression can leave family and friends feeling completely powerless to help. Patience, understanding, and support are necessary. Professional help should be sought if the patient talks of harming or killing him/herself.

It is often difficult to cope with the disruption caused by manic episodes. Information about the illness, and the need to take treatment and support should be provided. The patient should be gently steered away from social situations in which his/her anger, irritability, and expansive thinking can prove disruptive and difficult to manage.

People with bipolar disorder may need long-term support in order to get back to normal life. They will also need support to continue taking their medication for long periods in order to prevent further episodes of illness.

WHAT IS THE LONG-TERM OUTCOME OF BIPOLAR DISORDER?

Many people with bipolar disorder are able to lead normal lives. While the episodic nature of the illness can make life uncertain, the prophylactic medication can prevent episodes and helps many to go back to their jobs and take up responsibility. A minority of people with the disorder who do not respond to a single mood stabilizer can benefit from a combination of treatments. A few people with the condition are not able to get back to their old level of functioning.

You can discuss these and other issues with your doctor, nurse, or occupational therapist. You should feel free to clarify any doubts you have about disease and its treatment.

f. Information leaflet on depression and anxiety for patients and their families

WHAT ARE DEPRESSION AND ANXIETY?

Depression is a term used to describe persistent low mood, sadness, and misery. Anxiety is used to describe tension, stress, and uneasiness. We all feel fed up, miserable, uneasy, or sad at times. However, these feelings usually do not last longer than a week or two, and they do not interfere too much with our lives. Very often there is a reason for our low or anxious moods, but sometimes they just come out of the blue. We usually cope with them ourselves. We may have a chat with a friend but do not otherwise need any help. Someone is said to be significantly depressed or anxious, or suffering from depression or anxiety, when his/her feelings do not go away quickly and they interfere with his/her everyday life.

WHAT ARE THE SYMPTOMS OF DEPRESSION AND ANXIETY?

The symptoms of depression include feeling unhappy most of the time, loss of interest in life and the things one used to enjoy, finding it harder to make decisions, and feeling tired, lethargic, restless and agitated. Physical symptoms such as headaches can be distressing. Loss of appetite and weight, lack of confidence, feelings of hopeless, and loss of interest in sex can occur. Sleep is often disturbed and suicidal ideation can occur.

The symptoms of anxiety include worry, apprehension, muscle tension, fatigue, difficulty with concentration, irritability, and sleep disturbance. Episodic anxiety (called panic) or fear of certain situations (called phobia) may also occur. Often symptoms of depression and anxiety co-exist. The feelings of depression and anxiety are more unpleasant than the short episodes of unhappiness and tension that we all experience from time to time. They go on for much longer and can last for months rather than days or weeks.

WHAT ARE THE CAUSES OF DEPRESSION AND ANXIETY?

The causes of depression are many. The reason may seem obvious. It can be a disappointment, frustration, or losing something or someone important. It is normal to feel depressed after a distressing event, such as bereavement, a divorce, or losing a job. It can be after a physical illness, especially if it is chronic. Anxiety can be caused by increased stress and tensions that we face in our daily lives. We may spend time over the next few weeks or months thinking and talking about it. After a while we seem to come to terms with what has happened. But some of us get stuck in a depressed or anxious mood, which does not seem to lift.

Many people who drink too much alcohol become depressed. Women seem to get depressed more than men do. Women may be more likely to have the double stress of having to work and, at the same time, looking after children. The particular make-up of our body, experiences early in our life, or both may be responsible for depression and anxiety. Depression and anxiety can also run in families. If you have one parent who has become severely depressed, then you are about eight times more likely to become depressed yourself.

WHAT ARE THE COMMON LOCAL BELIEFS ABOUT CAUSATION?

Many people believe that depression and anxiety are a form of weakness or laziness that needs to be overcome. Supernatural causes, such as karma, black magic, evil spirits, sin, or punishment by God, are also suggested as causal, especially if the depression or anxiety is persistent. It is not the aim of this leaflet to dismiss such beliefs about causation, but to present a medical view of the condition. People seem to hold more than one belief about the cause. While we do not ask you to abandon your cultural beliefs, we would suggest that you also consider a medical model for depression and anxiety. Treatments from traditional faith healers and shamans can be employed in combination with medical and psychological treatment for the relief of suffering.

WHAT IS THE CLINICAL OUTCOME FOR PEOPLE WITH DEPRESSION AND ANXIETY?

Many people with depression and anxiety will recover. However, it can also persist in some people and cause significant distress. Persistent or severe depression can also lead to suicide. The sooner it is identified and managed, the better the outlook.

WHAT CAN I DO TO GET OUT OF DEPRESSION AND ANXIETY?

You can do many things to overcome depression and anxiety. These include:

- Talk to your friends and family. It often helps to go over the painful experience, to cry about it, and to talk things over with someone. This is part of nature's way of healing.
- Get regular exercise to keep physically fit.
- Try to take a good, balanced diet, even though you may not feel like eating. Fresh fruit and vegetables are particularly good.
- Avoid alcohol. Alcohol actually makes depression worse, and too much of it is also bad for your physical health and causes sleep disturbance.
- Try and revive your hobbies. They can help reduce the stress and tensions of life.
- If you are a religious person, consider regular prayer or visits to the local temple, church or mosque. Meditation is also helpful.
- Learning yoga or meditation is helpful in improving coping and in reducing anxiety and depression.
- Tackle the cause. If you think you know what is behind your depression, it can help to write down the problem, and then think of the things you could do to solve it.

When should I seek help?

- When your feelings of depression and anxiety are worse than usual, persistent, and do not seem to get any better
- When your feelings of depression and anxiety affect your work, interests, and feelings towards your family and friends
- If you find yourself feeling that life is not worth living, or that other people would be better off without you

It may be enough to talk things over with a relative or friend, who may be able to help you through the difficult situation in your life. If this does not seem to help, you probably need to talk it over with your doctor.

What is the treatment for depression and anxiety?

Most people with depression and anxiety can be treated by their family doctor. Depending on the symptoms, the severity of the symptoms, and the circumstances, the doctor may suggest some form of talking treatment (psychotherapy/counseling), antidepressant tablets, or both. Counseling is useful for mild depression and anxiety, and that precipitated by stress. Medication is indicated if the symptoms are severe and protracted. A certain class of medication, benzodiazepines (e.g. diazepam, lorazepam, or clonazepam) is best avoided as they are addictive.

Psychotherapy/counseling

Simply talking about your feelings can be helpful. If you have become depressed or anxious while suffering from a disability or caring for a relative, then sharing your experiences with others with similar problems may give you the support you need. Talking about recent bereavement is also useful. Talking with a trained counselor or therapist can sometimes be easier than talking to friends or relatives. There are many different sorts of psychotherapy available, some of which are very effective for people with mild to moderate depression and anxiety. Cognitive behavioral therapy helps people overcome the negative thoughts that can sometimes be the cause of depression. Interpersonal therapies are helpful if you find it difficult to get on with other people. However, talking treatments do take time to work. Counseling sessions usually last about an hour and the course of therapy usually lasts from 5 to 10 sessions. These sessions are usually held once a week, although you can meet your counselor more frequently, if required.

Antidepressants

If your depression is severe or has been persistent, your doctor may suggest that you take antidepressant medication. These medicines relieve depression and anxiety by increasing the function of chemical messengers in the brain, such as serotonin and noradrenaline. Although these medicines may help you feel less anxious and agitated, they are not tranquillizers and are not addictive. They help people with depression to feel and cope better. However, while sleep may improve immediately, these medicines usually take 2–3 weeks to relieve depression. Like all medicines, antidepressants also have minor side-effects. These are usually mild and tend to decrease with time. The older antidepressants can cause a dry mouth, sedation, and constipation, while the newer ones may cause nausea.

How long will I have to take medication?

Most doctors will suggest that you take medication for about six months after you recover from your depression and anxiety.

You can discuss these and other issues with your doctor, nurse, or occupational therapist. You should feel free to clarify any doubts you have about depression and anxiety and their treatment.

g. Information leaflet for people with persistent physical symptoms and anxiety about their health

Many people who report distressing physical symptoms present to GPs with persistent worries about their health.

WHAT ARE THE COMMON PHYSICAL SYMPTOM PRESENTATIONS?

People often present to general and family physicians with a wide variety of physical symptoms. Physicians with their clinical skill and currently available technology are able to identify specific pathology in a proportion of their patients. Many other patients, however, have persistent symptoms without any identifiable abnormalities, despite the distressing nature of their complaints.

Such physical symptoms include tiredness, lethargy, fatigue, or specific worries about symptoms such as headache or chest pain. Other patterns include irritable bowel syndrome, which has a complex pattern of diarrhea and abdominal cramps.

WHAT IS HEALTH ANXIETY?

Health anxiety is a label used to describe clinical presentations of people with or without physical symptoms, who may or may not have diagnosable medical diseases, who present with a preoccupation about having or acquiring a serious illness. They have a high level of anxiety about health, are easily alarmed about their personal health status, and frequently seek medical examination, intervention, and reassurance.

WHAT IS THE PREVALENCE OF SUCH PRESENTATIONS?

Such presentations are commonly seen in about a third or a fourth of people attending primary care and general medical facilities. Many surveys have documented an increase in such presentations over time. This increase in prevalence is correlated with an increase in the medicalization of distress in society. The breakdown of traditional family, social, and community support and the increase in the use of the internet make anxious people to selectively focus on the most serious explanation for symptoms, even though these may be very uncommon. Such anxiety is often very disabling and is associated with long-term morbidity, increased sick leave, and absence from work.

CAN PEOPLE WITH PHYSICAL PRESENTATIONS HAVE PSYCHIATRIC DISORDERS?

The general population expects doctors to manage physical complaints rather than psychological and social distress. Consequently, patients presenting to general medical settings with psychiatric and psychosocial problems often report somatic complaints. Only a proportion of people with such presentations will have diagnosable psychiatric disorders such as anxiety and depression. These presentations are mild, mixed, and frequently associated with psychosocial adversity.

WHAT HAPPENS TO PATIENTS WHO DO NOT GET HELP FROM PHYSICIANS?

The inability of physicians to identify physical causes for somatic symptoms and manage such presentations often results in the physician downplaying their importance and ignoring the patient's distress. Consequently, many patients are often dissatisfied with the medical consultation and the care and treatment that they receive. Such dissatisfaction results in patients visiting many doctors and hospitals, shopping for different treatments and solutions.

WHAT IS THE CLINICAL OUTCOME FOR PEOPLE WITH PERSISTENT PHYSICAL SYMPTOMS?

Many people with physical symptoms and health anxiety will recover. The absence of specific medical explanations and particular solutions to their problems means that they receive only symptomatic therapies, which can reduce their symptoms. The majority are able to manage with symptomatic treatments and get on with their lives. Only a small minority of people with such presentations continue to focus on their illness and shop for medical solutions. Long-term reduction in symptoms, distress, and disability may require non-medical strategies.

WHAT CAN I DO TO OBTAIN RELIEF?

You can do many things to overcome your physical symptoms and anxiety about your health. These include:

- Talk to your friends and family. It often helps to go over the difficult or painful experience, to cry about it, and to talk things over with someone. This is part of nature's way of healing.
- Get regular exercise. Going out of the house for walks can be helpful. Keeping physically fit through exercise or yoga are options.
- Try to take a good, balanced diet, even though you may not feel like eating. Fresh fruit and vegetables are particularly good.
- Avoid alcohol. Alcohol actually makes depression and anxiety worse, and too much of it is bad for your physical health and may cause sleep disturbance.
- Try and revive your hobbies. They can help reduce the stress and tensions of life.
- If you are a religious person, consider regular prayer or visits to the local temple, church, or mosque.
- Learning yoga or meditation is helpful in improving coping and in reducing anxiety and depression.

- Tackle the cause. If you think you know what is behind your depression, it can help to write down the problem and then think of the things you could do to solve it.

WHEN SHOULD I SEEK HELP?

- When your feelings of depression and anxiety are worse than usual, persistent, and do not seem to get any better.
- When your feelings of depression and anxiety affect your work, interests, and feelings towards your family and friends.
- If you find yourself feeling that life is not worth living, or that other people would be better off without you.

It may be enough to talk things over with a relative or friend, who may be able to help you through the difficult situation in your life. If this does not seem to help, you probably need to talk it over with your doctor.

WHAT IS THE TREATMENT FOR DEPRESSION AND ANXIETY?

While people with physical symptoms are usually prescribed medication and non-drug solutions for reducing their symptoms, their family doctor can treat those with anxiety and depression. Depending on the symptoms, the severity of the symptoms and the circumstances, the doctor may suggest some form of talking treatment (psychotherapy/counseling), antidepressant tablets, or both. Counseling is useful for mild depression and anxiety, and that precipitated by stress. Medication is indicated if the symptoms are severe and protracted. A certain class of medication, benzodiazepines (e.g. diazepam, lorazepam, and clonazepam), is best avoided, as they are addictive.

PSYCHOTHERAPY/COUNSELING

Simply talking about your feelings can be helpful. If you have become depressed or anxious while suffering from a disability or caring for a relative, then sharing your experiences with others with similar problems may give you the support you need. Talking about recent bereavement is also useful. Talking with a trained counselor or therapist can sometimes be easier than talking to friends or relatives. There are many different sorts of psychotherapy available, some of which are very effective for people with mild to moderate depression and anxiety. Cognitive behavioral therapy helps people overcome the negative thoughts that can sometimes be the cause of depression. Interpersonal therapies are helpful if you find it difficult to get on with other people. However, talking treatments do take time to work. Counseling sessions usually last about an hour and the course of therapy usually lasts from five to ten sessions. These sessions are usually held once a week, although you can meet your counselor more frequently, if required.

MEDICATION

Your physician may prescribe medication for the symptomatic relief of your suffering. If your depression is severe or has been persistent, your doctor may suggest that you take antidepressant medication. These medicines relieve depression and anxiety by increasing the function of chemical messengers in the brain, such as serotonin and noradrenaline. Although these medicines may help you feel less anxious and agitated, they are not tranquilizers and are not addictive. They help people with depression to feel and cope better. However, while sleep may improve immediately, these medicines usually take 2–3 weeks to relieve depression. Like all medicines, antidepressants also have minor side-effects. These are usually mild and tend to decrease with time. The older antidepressants can cause a dry mouth, sedation, and constipation, while the newer ones may cause nausea. Most doctors will suggest that you take medication for about six months after you recover from your depression and anxiety.

You can discuss these and other issues with your doctor, nurse, or occupational therapist. You should feel free to clarify any doubts you have.

h. Marriage and the law: Information for people with mental illness

CAN PEOPLE WHO HAVE HAD A MENTAL ILLNESS GET MARRIED?

Yes, people with mental illness can get married.

ARE THERE ANY PRECONDITIONS FOR GETTING MARRIED FOR PEOPLE WHO HAVE HAD A MENTAL ILLNESS?

The general preconditions are:

- The symptoms of the illness should be under control with treatment.
- The person should be able to look after him/herself and be able to work either in the home if he/she plans to be a homemaker or outside the home if he/she plans to have a career and earn a living.
- The person should understand the nature of marriage and its implications and obligations.
- The person should be able to give valid consent for the marriage.
- The future bride or bridegroom and her/his family should be told about the illness and its treatment.

WHY SHOULD THESE PRECONDITIONS BE MET BEFORE MARRIAGE?

Marriage, per se, can be stressful for some people and hence, it is better to get married after the symptoms of illness are completely controlled with treatment. Holding a job or being able to do the household work implies that you have reached a good level of functioning. The person should also understand the implications of marriage and be able to consent to the contract. The fiancée/fiancé and his/her family should be told about the illness and its treatment as many problems arise if we deceive them by withholding such information.

WHAT ARE THE LAWS RELATED TO MARRIAGE IN INDIA?

There are many laws related to marriage in India. These include:
- The Hindu Marriage Act, 1955 applies to Hindus, Buddhists, Jains, and Sikhs.
- Muslim Personal Law, 1937 applies to Muslims.
- The Indian Christian Marriage Act, 1872 applies to Christians
- The Parsi Marriage and Divorce Act, 1936 applies to those who are Parsi.
- The Special Marriage Act, 1954 can be employed if you prefer a civil marriage.

WHICH LAWS WILL BE APPLICABLE TO ME?

The laws related to marriage which apply to you depend on which religion you follow and on the marriage ceremony you choose. If you choose a religious ceremony, then the laws related to marriage under that religion will apply. If the person you intend to marry follows another religion or if both of you prefer a civil marriage, then your marriage can be conducted under the Special Marriage Act, 1954.

HOW SHOULD THESE LAWS BE VIEWED?

Although there have been a few amendments to some laws related to marriage and divorce, most laws are at least 50 years old. The understanding of mental illness has changed since then. Mental illness is not one category but many. The terms related to mental illness employed in drafting these laws are not employed for diagnosis these days. Many effective treatments are also now available. The general prognosis of mental disorders is very much better now than it was when these laws were made. So while these laws apply to the marriage contract, recent judgments of the Supreme Court of India suggest that mental illness, per se, does not disqualify one from marriage or other contracts.

WHAT WILL HAPPEN IF I DO NOT DISCLOSE MY MENTAL ILLNESS TO MY FIANCÉE/FIANCÉ?

Concealment of the fact that you have/had a mental illness leads to a breakdown of trust and strains the marital relationship. This will become evident if your spouse notices that you are taking medication, or if you have a relapse of the illness. Concealment of the fact that you have/had a mental illness is recognized by the courts as "deception/fraud" and can be a ground for annulling the marriage. Concealment of such facts often results in a legal/court case, and adds additional stress and financial burden.

WILL DISCLOSURE ABOUT MY MENTAL ILLNESS REDUCE MY CHANCE OF GETTING MARRIED?

While this is possible, it may be better to marry someone who will understand you and your illness, and its treatment. A supportive spouse will also aid in your recovery and in coping.

IS MENTAL ILLNESS, PER SE, A GROUND FOR DIVORCE?

While laws related to marriage state that mental illness is a ground for annulment of marriage/divorce, the Supreme Court of India has recently ruled that mental illness, per se, is not a ground for divorce. However, often the spouses of people with mental illness can and do go to court seeking separation/divorce.

WHAT ARE THE GROUNDS FOR DIVORCE IF ONE PARTNER IN A MARRIAGE HAS A MENTAL ILLNESS?

The development of mental illness after marriage per se is not a ground for divorce. However, the following will support arguments for annulment of marriage/divorce:

- deception and concealment of mental illness prior to marriage
- inability to give valid consent for the procedure

- inability to live up to the roles and responsibilities of marriage because of mental illness
- mental or physical cruelty
- unconsummated marriage or erectile dysfunction.

WHAT ARE THE PROCEDURES RELATED TO JUDICIAL SEPARATION, DIVORCE, MAINTENANCE, AND CHILD CUSTODY?

These procedures are complex and you should contact your lawyer for the details. You can also contact the legal aid services in your district court and they will be able to give you advice free of cost.

You can discuss these and other issues with your doctor. You should feel free to clarify any doubts you have about marriage, the laws, and their implications. You should also discuss the issues related to your illness, its treatment, and prognosis.

i. Information leaflet on making a WILL for people with mental illness

This leaflet provides details on how a person with mental illness can make a WILL in order that he/she can distribute his property and wealth after his/her death.

What is a WILL?

A WILL is a document in which a person specifies the method to be applied in the management and distribution of his estate, property, or wealth after his/her death.

What are the basic requirements to be able to make a WILL?

The basic requirements for making a WILL are:

- The person must know the nature and extent of his/her assets and property.
- The person must know who are his/her natural heirs.
- The person should know the significance of a WILL and that he/she is making a WILL.

The capacity to make a WILL is also called "testamentary capacity" and implies that a person has the mental competence to make a WILL.

Can people who have had a mental illness make a WILL?

Yes, people with mental illness can make a WILL.

Are there any other preconditions for making a WILL for people who have had a mental illness?

No, there are no other preconditions for making a WILL. If the person satisfies the basic requirements for making a WILL, then he/she is eligible to make a WILL. The law does not discriminate against people with mental illness in particular, provided that they satisfy the basic requirements that are applicable to people without mental illness.

What happens when you do not make a WILL?

When a person dies without having made a WILL, he/she is said to have died intestate. His property is then inherited by his/her legal heirs in accordance with the law of inheritance applicable to him/her. Legal heirs generally include close family members, such as one's spouse, children, parents, brothers, and sisters.

WHY SHOULD PEOPLE MAKE A WILL?

There are many reasons for and advantages of making a WILL. These include:

- It will allow the person to dispose of property according to his/her wish.
- It will prevent the confusion and conflict that often arise in the absence of a WILL. Disputes can be prevented and easily resolved if there is a WILL.
- It allows the person to appoint a guardian for children below 18 years of age.
- It will allow taking into account special needs, such as those of children with physical and mental handicaps and illness.

WHY SHOULD PEOPLE WITH MENTAL ILLNESS MAKE A WILL?

Many disputes can occur after the death of the person. Often WILLs are challenged on the basis of the fact that the person had been diagnosed to have a mental illness, was on treatment, did not have the testamentary capacity, or was deceived into writing the WILL. It is very difficult to support the contention that the person had/did not have the testamentary capacity after his/her death and this leads to prolonged legal battles. A certification of testamentary capacity by the psychiatrist, the writing of a WILL, and getting it witnessed and notarized/registered will prevent such confusion.

WHAT ARE THE LAWS RELATED TO SUCCESSION IN INDIA?

The Indian Succession Act, 1925 is the relevant law in India. However, for Hindus, Buddhists, Jains and Sikhs, the laws of inheritance have been codified in the Hindu Succession Act, 1956. Muslims have their own law based on their religious texts, and the law differs for Shias and Sunnis.

WHAT ARE THE STEPS IN MAKING A WILL?

- List your assets.
- Make provision for estate/inheritance tax, if applicable.
- List your beneficiaries.
- Decide on the set allocations to the beneficiaries.
- Decide on the executors.
- Decide on a guardian if you have a child below 18 years of age.
- Select an estate guardian or a trustee if you want the parental duties separate from managing the property.
- Decide where to keep your WILL.
- Inform all your loved ones about the location of the WILL.

ARE THERE ANY SPECIAL LEGAL FORMALITIES REQUIRED TO MAKE THE WILL LEGALLY VALID?

You need to execute the WILL after you have written it. This includes the following steps:

- The WILL has to be signed by the required witnesses, who are not beneficiaries.
- The WILL has to be notarized/registered.

Should you update your WILL?

Once people make a WILL, they will put it in a safe deposit box/place. However, there are many reasons to review and update your WILL and these include new births or adoptions, marriage and divorce, death of named beneficiaries, and marked increase in assets. The passage of time is reason enough. You should review your WILL every 3 to 5 years.

What is the procedure after death to implement the WILL?

The WILL has to be probated. A probate is the process of transferring the estate of the deceased to the beneficiary. It also involves the process of identifying, listing, accounting, and appraisal of the deceased's property, and payment of taxes and creditors. This is usually done in a probate court. This process is easy if the WILL was written clearly and with all the necessary details.

What are the details of the procedures involved

You should contact your lawyer for details. You can also contact the legal aid services in your district court and they will be able to give you advice free of cost.

You can discuss these and other issues with your doctor. You should feel free to clarify any doubts you have about the WILL, and the laws and their implications.

Section VIII

Bibliography

Index

Bibliography

The material in this book has been developed over many years based on our previous publications in the field. These have been published on different e-learning websites, in national and international journals, and in books. The list includes the following:

The following modules were published on the e-learning website of the Christian Medical College, Vellore (Kuruvilla A and Jacob KS, 2007–08): (i) Introduction; (ii) Delirium; (iii) Dementia; (iv) Alcohol dependence; (v) Psychosis; (vi) Medically unexplained symptoms; (vii) Attempted suicide and suicidal risk; (vii) Nocturnal enuresis; (viii) Temper tantrums; (ix) Basic medication management; and (x) Basic communication and counseling skills.

The following modules were developed for the website of the Tamil Nadu Special Hospital Project (Kuruvilla A and Jacob KS, 2007–08): (i) Introduction; (ii) The management of delirium; (iii) The management of dementia; (iv) The management of substance dependence; (v) The management of psychosis; (vi) The management of medically unexplained symptoms; (vii) The management of attempted suicide and suicidal risk; (vii) Nocturnal enuresis in children; (viii) Temper tantrums in children; (ix) Basic psychotropic medication management; and (x) Counseling skills.

The patient information leaflets were developed for use in the Department of Psychiatry, Christian Medical College, Vellore, Tamil Nadu, India.

The following articles have appeared in national and international journals:

1. Kumar DS, Jacob KS. Managing a violent patient. *Natl Med J India* 1994;7:140–2.
2. Kuruvilla A, Pothen M, Philip K, Braganza D, Joseph A, Jacob KS. The validation of the Tamil version of the 12-item General Health Questionnaire. *Indian J Psychiatry* 1999;41:217–21.
3. Manoharam E, Jebaraj P, Jacob KS. Diagnosis and management of panic disorder in medical practice. *Natl Med J India* 2000;13:204–6.
4. Braganza D, Kuruvilla A, Joseph A, Jacob KS. Criteria for neurasthenia. *Aust N Z J Psychiatry* 2000;34:340.
5. Jacob KS. Basic counselling skills for medical practice. *Natl Med J India* 2000;13: 25–8.
6. Sathyaseelan M, Seema P, Maret J, Saravanan B, Ezhilrasu P, Jacob KS. Patient perspectives on psychosis. *Indian J Psychiatry* 2001;43(S):72.
7. Manoharam E, John KR, Joseph A, Jacob KS. Psychiatric morbidity, patient perspectives of illness and factors associated with poor medication compliance among the tuberculous in Vellore, South India. *Indian J Tuberculosis* 2001;48:77–80.
8. Nambi SK, Prasad J, Singh D, Abraham V, Kuruvilla A, Jacob KS. Explanatory models and common mental disorders among subjects with unexplained somatic symptoms in a primary care facility in Tamil Nadu. *Natl Med J India* 2002;15:331–5.
9. Pothen M, Kuruvilla A, Philip K, Joseph A, Jacob KS. Common mental disorders among primary care attenders in Vellore, South India: Nature, prevalence and risk factors. *Int J Soc Psychiatry* 2003;49:119–25.
10. Nambi SK, Prasad J, Singh D, Abraham V, Kuruvilla A, Jacob KS. Explanatory models and common mental disorders among subjects with unexplained somatic symptoms in a primary care facility in Tamil Nadu. *Natl Med J India* 2002;15:331–5.
11. Jebaraj P, Jebaraj I, Sunderaraj GD, Korula RJ, Jacob KS. Common mental disorders in

subjects with chronic low back pain in Vellore, South India: Nature, prevalence and risk factors. *Indian J Psychol Med* 2003;26:24–7.

12. Jacob KS. Misunderstanding depression. *Natl Med J India* 2003;16:270–2.

13. Koshy S, Jacob KS. Management of unexplained somatic symptoms in general and dental hospital settings. *Indian J Psychiatry* 2004;6:382–3.

14. Jacob KS. Teaching medical students to diagnose depression: A different approach. *Natl Med J India* 2004;17:261–5.

15. Jacob KS. A simple protocol to manage unexplained somatic symptoms in medical practice. *Natl Med J India* 2004;17:326–8.

16. Gopalakrishnan R, Kurian S, Jacob KS. Psychological management of erectile dysfunction in primary care. *Natl Med J India* 2005;18:274.

17. Jacob KS. The diagnosis and management of depression and anxiety in primary care: The need for a different framework. *Postgrad Med J* 2006;82:836–9.

18. Jacob KS. The cultures of depression. *Natl Med J India* 2006;19:218–20.

19. Kuruvilla A, Jacob KS. The management of psychosis in primary care. *Natl Med J India* 2006;19:325–9.

20. Jacob KS. Major depression: A review of the concept and the diagnosis. *Adv Psychiatr Treatment* 2009;15:279–85.

21. Jacob KS. Bridging the disease-illness divide in modern medicine. *Natl Med J India* 2009;22:320–2.

22. Vijayprasad G, Mathew AJ, Radhakrishnan S, Arulappan N, Christa JA, Jacob KS. Knowledge, attitude and practice related to medically unexplained symptoms among physicians. *Natl Med J India* 2009;22:279.

22. John A, Barman A, Bal D, Chandy G, Samuel J, Thokchom M, Joy N, Vijaykumar P, Thapa S, Singh V, Raghava V, Seshadri T, Jacob KS, Balraj V. Hazardous alcohol use in rural south India: Nature, prevalence and risk factors. *Natl Med J India* 2009;22;123–5.

23. Jacob KS. Alcohol and public health policies in India. *Natl Med J India* 2010;23:224–5.

24. Jacob KS, Kuruvilla A. Psychotherapy across cultures: The form–content dichotomy. *Clin Psychology Psychotherapy* 2012;19:91–5.

25. Jacob KS. Repackaging mental health programmes for low and middle-income countries. *Indian J Psychiatry* 2011;53:195–8.

26. Jacob KS. Alcohol and public health policies in India. *The Globe* 2011;1:15–18.

27. Jacob KS. Chasing biological mirages, ignoring contextual reality. *Indian J Soc Psychiatry* 2012;28:1–2;15–19.

28. Jacob KS. Patient experience and psychiatric discourse. *The Psychiatrist* 2012;36:414–17.

29. Rao TSS, Gopalakrishnan R, Kuruvilla A, Jacob KS. Social determinants of sexual health. *Indian J Psychiatry* 2012;54:105–7.

30. Duba AS, Rajkumar AP, Prince MJ, Jacob KS. Determinants of disability among elderly in a rural south Indian community: Need to study local issues and contexts. *Int Psychogeriatrics* 2012;24:333–41.

31. 24. Varghese KM, Bansal R, Kekre AN, Jacob KS. Sexual dysfunction among young married women in south India. *Int Urogynecology J* 2012;23:1771–4.

32. 25. Kuruvilla A, Jacob KS. Perceptions about anxiety, depression and somatization in general medical settings: A qualitative study from Vellore, South India. *Natl Med J India* 2012;25:332–5.

33. Jacob KS. Depression: A major public health problem in need of a multi-sectoral response. *Indian J Med Res* 2012;136:537–9.

34. Jacob KS. Dementia: Toward contextual understanding. *Int Psychogeriatrics* 2012:24:1703–7.

35. Kim, S-M, Rifkin S, John SM, Jacob KS. Nature, prevalence, and risk factors of alcohol use in urban slum in southern India. *Natl Med J India* 2013;26:203–9.

36. Jacob KS. Diagnostic and Statistical Manual-5: No revolutionary road. *Natl Med J India* 2013;26:255–7.
37. Jacob KS. Psychosocial adversity and mental illness: Differentiating distress, contextualizing diagnosis. *Indian J Psychiatry* 2013;55:106–10.
38. Jacob KS. Depression: Disease, distress and double bind. *Australian NZ J Psychiatry* 2013;47:304–8.
39. Jacob KS. Employing psychotherapy across cultures and contexts. *Indian J Psychol Med* 2013;35:323–5.
40. Jacob KS. Depression: Identifying, managing and preventing disease and distress. *Christian Med J India* 2013;28:12–14.
41. Viswanathan SA, Prasad JH, Jacob KS, Kuruvilla A. Sexual function in women in rural Tamil Nadu: Disease, dysfunction, distress and norms. *Natl Med J India* 2014;27:4–8.
42. Nongrum R, Thomas E, Lionel J, Jacob KS. Domestic violence as a risk factor for maternal depression and neonatal outcomes: a hospital-based cohort study. *Indian J Psychol Med* 2014;36:179–81.
43. Thangadurai P, Gopalakrishnan R, Kuruvilla A, Jacob KS. Sexual dysfunction in secondary care in South India: Nature, prevalence, clinical features and explanatory models. *Natl Med J India* 2014;27:198–201.
44. Jacob KS, Kallivayalil RA, Mallik AK, Gupta N, Trivedi JK, Gangadhar BN, Praveenlal K, Vahia V, Rao TSS. Diagnostic and Statistical Manual-5: Position paper of the Indian Psychiatric Society. *Indian J Psychiatry* 2013;55:12–30.
45. Jacob KS. Dementia: Comparing local and international data, perspectives and conclusion. *Natl Med J India* 2014;27:95–8.
46. Jacob KS. DSM-5 and culture: The need to move towards a shared model of care within a more equal patient–physician partnership. *Asian J Psychiatry* 2014;7:89–91.
47. Jacob KS. DSM-5 and dementia: Fine print, finer points. *Indian J Psychiatry* 2014;56:117–20.
48. Jacob KS, Patel V. Classification of mental disorders: A global mental health perspective. *Lancet* 2014;383:1433–5.
49. Jacob KS. The challenge of medical diagnosis: A primer on principles, probability, process and pitfalls. *Natl Med J India* 2015;28:24–28.
50. Jacob KS. Mental illness: Diverse perspectives, partial truths, imperfect solutions. *MFC Bulletin* 2015;363/364:22–25.
51. Jacob KS. Recovery model of mental illness: A complementary approach to psychiatric care. *Indian J Psychol Med* 2015;37:117–19.
52. Jacob KS. Mental distress, disease, diagnosis and treatment: The bigger questions. *Economic and Political Weekly* 2015;L:17.
53. Jacob KS. Mental Health Care: New tactics, failed strategy. *Economic and Political Weekly* 2015;51:15–18.
54. Jacob KS. Patient experience and the psychiatric discourse: Attempting to bridge incommensurable worlds. *Indian J Psychiatry* 2015:57:423–6.
55. Jacob KS. Post-traumatic stress disorder: Psychiatric management, atonement and justice. *Natl Med J India* 2015;28:198–200.

The following chapters have been published in books:
1. Raghuthaman G, Jacob KS, Ranjith G. The diagnosis and management of delirium and dementia. In: Bhugra D, Ranjith G, Patel V (eds). *Handbook of psychiatry: A South Asian perspective*. New Delhi: Byword Viva Publishers; 2005.
2. Dutta SS, Kumar S, Jacob KS. Clinical features of dementia. In: Kar N, Jolly D, Misra B (eds). *Handbook of dementia*. Hyderabad: Paras Medical Publishers; 2005.

3. Jacob KS. Liaison psychiatry. In: Verghese A, Abraham A (eds). *Introduction to psychiatry.* Chennai: ELS Publishers; 2007.

4. Jacob KS. Reclaiming primary care: Managing depression and anxiety in a different framework. In: Zachariah A, Srivats R. Tharu S (eds). *Towards a critical medical practice: Reflections on the dilemmas of medical culture today.* Orient Blackswan, New Delhi; 2010: pp311–19.

5. Jacob KS. PTSD, DSM and India: A critique. In: Zachariah A, Srivats R. Tharu S (eds). *Towards a critical medical practice: Reflections on the dilemmas of medical culture today.* New Delhi: Orient Blackswan; 2010: pp57–68.

6. Jacob KS, Prince M, Goldberg D. Confirmatory factor analysis of common mental disorders. In: Goldberg DP, Kendler KS, Sirovatka P, Regier DA (eds). *Diagnostic issues in depression and generalized anxiety disorders: Refining the research agenda for DSM-V.* American Psychiatric Association: Arlington; 2010.

7. Kuruvilla A, Jacob KS. Psychosocial issues in HIV and AIDS. In: Temesgen Z (ed). *Fundamentals of global HIV medicine.* American Academy of HIV Medicine; 2010.

8. Kuruvilla A, Jacob KS. Stigma in mental illness. In: Bhugra D, Gopinath R, Patel V, Jagan NC (eds). *Handbook of Psychiatry: A South Asian Perspective,* Edition 2. Anshan Publishing; 2010.

9. Jacob KS. Indian psychiatry and the classification of psychiatric disorders. In: TSS Rao (ed). *Indian research in psychiatry: A journey of six decades.* Mysore: Indian Psychiatric Society; 2010: pp213–23.

10. Kuruvilla A, Jacob KS. Public mental health and India. In: *Public mental health: An evolving field.* New Delhi: Ministry of Health, Government of India; 2011.

11. Jacob KS, Kuruvilla A. Culture and its impact on diagnosis and management of mental disorders: The cultural formulation. In: TSS Rao (ed). *Psychiatric training in India: Training and training centres.* Mysore: Indian Psychiatric Society; 2011.

12. Kuruvilla A, Jacob KS. Mental health resources in South Asia. In: Trivedi JK, Tripathi A (eds). *Mental health in South Asia: Ethics, resources, programs and legislation.* Edition 2. International Library of Ethics, Law and the New Medicine, Vol 58 Springer, 2015; pp191–220.

13. Jacob KS. Changing cultures within medicine. In: Kallolicckal V. (ed). *Medicine and Society.* Department of History, Maharaja's College, Ernakulam; 2012: pp17–21.

14. Kuruvilla A, Ravindran A, Jacob KS. Psychiatric emergencies in medical conditions. In: Thara R, Vijaykumar L (eds). *Emergencies in psychiatry in low- and middle-income countries.* Byword Books, Delhi; 2012: pp136–54.

15. Jacob KS. Gay rights and bigotry: Reflection on the relationship between science, medicine, psychiatry, society, religion and the Church. In: Zachariah G (ed). *Church and homophobia: Re-imagining church as rainbow community.* CISRS and ISPCK; 2014.

Index